T0226537

Hot Topics in Dermatology

Editor

KENNETH J. TOMECKI

DERMATOLOGIC CLINICS

www.derm.theclinics.com

Consulting Editor
BRUCE H. THIERS

January 2019 • Volume 37 • Number 1

ELSEVIER

1600 John F. Kennedy Boulevard • Suite 1800 • Philadelphia, Pennsylvania, 19103-2899

http://www.theclinics.com

DERMATOLOGIC CLINICS Volume 37, Number 1
January 2019 ISSN 0733-8635, ISBN-13: 978-0-323-65497-5

Editor: Jessica McCool
Developmental Editor: Sara Watkins

Dermatologic Clinics (ISSN 0733-8635) is published quarterly by Elsevier Inc., 360 Park Avenue South, New York, NY 10010-1710. Months of publication are January, April, July, and October. Business and editorial offices: 1600 John F. Kennedy Blvd., Suite 1800, Philadelphia, PA 19103-2899. Customer service office: 11830 Westline Drive, St. Louis, MO 63146. Periodicals postage paid at New York, NY, and additional mailing offices. Subscription prices are USD 404.00 per year for US individuals, USD 736.00 per year for US institutions, USD 456.00 per year for Canadian individuals, USD 898.00 per year for Canadian institutions, USD 510.00 per year for international individuals, USD 898.00 per year for international institutions, USD 100.00 per year for US students/residents, and USD 240.00 per year for Canadian and international students/residents. International air speed delivery is included in all *Clinics* subscription prices. All prices are subject to change without notice. **POSTMASTER:** Send address changes to *Dermatologic Clinics*, Elsevier Health Sciences Division, Subscription Customer Service, 3251 Riverport Lane, Maryland Heights, MO 63043. **Customer Service: 1-800-654-2452 (U.S. and Canada); 314-447-8871 (outside U.S. and Canada). Fax: 314-447-8029. E-mail: journalscustomerservice-usa@elsevier.com (for print support); journalsonlinesupport-usa@elsevier.com (for online support).**

Reprints. For copies of 100 or more, of articles in this publication, please contact the Commercial Reprints Department, Elsevier Inc., 360 Park Avenue South, New York, New York 10010-1710. Tel.: 212-633-3874; Fax: 212-633-3820; Email: reprints@elsevier.com.

The *Dermatologic Clinics* is covered in *MEDLINE/PubMed (Index Medicus)*, *Current Contents/Clinical Medicine, Excerpta Medica, Chemical Abstracts,* and *ISI/BIOMED.*

Contributors

CONSULTING EDITOR

BRUCE H. THIERS, MD
Professor and Chairman Emeritus, Department
of Dermatology and Dermatologic Surgery,
Medical University of South Carolina,
Charleston, South Carolina, USA

EDITOR

KENNETH J. TOMECKI, MD
Department of Dermatology, Cleveland Clinic,
Cleveland, Ohio, USA

AUTHORS

HILARY E. BALDWIN, MD
Medical Director, The Acne Treatment and
Research Center of the DermGroup, Morristown,
New Jersey; Clinical Associate Professor of
Dermatology, Rutgers Robert Wood Johnson
Medical Center, Piscataway, New Jersey, USA

ANTHONY V. BENEDETTO, DO, FACP
Clinical Professor, Department of
Dermatology, Perelman School of Medicine,
University of Pennsylvania, Dermatologic
SurgiCenter, Philadelphia, Pennsylvania, USA

DAVID E. COHEN, MD, MPH
Charles C. and Dorothea E. Harris Professor of
Dermatology and Vice Chair for Clinical Affairs,
The Ronald O. Perelman Department of
Dermatology, NYU School of Medicine,
New York, New York, USA

LINDSEY COLLINS, MD
Assistant Professor, Department of
Dermatology, The University of Oklahoma
Health Sciences Center, Oklahoma City,
Oklahoma, USA

ADRIAN CUELLAR-BARBOZA, MD
Department of Dermatology, University
Hospital "Dr. José E. González," UANL,
Monterrey, Mexico

ZOE DIANA DRAELOS, MD
Dermatology Consulting Services, PLLC,
High Point, North Carolina, USA

LAWRENCE F. EICHENFIELD, MD
Division of Pediatric and Adolescent
Dermatology, Rady Children's Hospital,
Departments of Dermatology and Pediatrics,
University of California, San Diego School of
Medicine, San Diego, California,
USA

ANTHONY P. FERNANDEZ, MD, PhD
Assistant Clinical Professor, Cleveland Clinic
Lerner College of Medicine, W.D. Steck Chair
of Clinical Dermatology, Director of Medical
and Inpatient Dermatology, Staff
Dermatologist and Dermatopathologist,
Departments of Dermatology and Pathology,
Cleveland Clinic, Cleveland, Ohio,
USA

ADAM FRIEDMAN, MD, FAAD
Professor, Department of Dermatology,
George Washington Medical Faculty
Associates, Department of Dermatology,
George Washington School of Medicine and
Health Sciences, Washington, DC,
USA

JESUS ALBERTO CARDENAS-DE LA GARZA, MD
Department of Dermatology, University Hospital "Dr. José E. González," UANL, Monterrey, Mexico

ALLISON M. HAN, BA
Division of Pediatric and Adolescent Dermatology, Rady Children's Hospital, Departments of Dermatology and Pediatrics, University of California, San Diego School of Medicine, San Diego, California, USA

SOTONYE IMADOJEMU, MD, MBE
Department of Dermatology, Harvard Medical School, Harvard University, Boston, MA, USA

HEE J. KIM, MD
Clinical Research Fellow, Department of Dermatology, Icahn School of Medicine at Mount Sinai, New York, New York, USA

AYAN KUSARI, MA
Division of Pediatric and Adolescent Dermatology, Rady Children's Hospital, Departments of Dermatology and Pediatrics, University of California, San Diego School of Medicine, San Diego, California, USA

MARK G. LEBWOHL, MD
Professor, Chairman, Department of Dermatology, Icahn School of Medicine at Mount Sinai, New York, New York, USA

JUSTIN W. MARSON, BA
MS4, Rutgers Robert Wood Johnson Medical School, Piscataway, New Jersey, USA

JOSE DARIO MARTINEZ, MD
Department of Internal Medicine, University Hospital "Dr. José E. González," UANL, Monterrey, Mexico

EMILY C. MILAM, MD
The Ronald O. Perelman Department of Dermatology, NYU School of Medicine, New York, New York, USA

ANDREW QUINN, MD
Resident, Department of Dermatology, The University of Oklahoma Health Sciences Center, Oklahoma City, Oklahoma, USA

AZAM QURESHI, BA
Research Fellow, Department of Dermatology, George Washington Medical Faculty Associates, Washington, DC, USA

MISHA ROSENBACH, MD
Departments of Dermatology and Internal Medicine, Perelman School of Medicine, University of Pennsylvania, Philadelphia, PA, USA

DAVID SCHAIRER, MD
Division of Pediatric and Adolescent Dermatology, Rady Children's Hospital, Departments of Dermatology and Pediatrics, University of California, San Diego School of Medicine, San Diego, California, USA

THOMAS STASKO, MD
Professor, Chair, Department of Dermatology, The University of Oklahoma Health Sciences Center, Oklahoma City, Oklahoma, USA

ELISABETH HAMELIN TRACEY, MD
Resident, Department of Dermatology, Dermatology and Plastic Surgery Institute, Cleveland Clinic Foundation, Cleveland, Ohio, USA

ALOK VIJ, MD
Staff Dermatologist, Department of Dermatology, Dermatology and Plastic Surgery Institute, Cleveland Clinic Foundation, Clinical Assistant Professor of Medicine, Cleveland Clinic Lerner College of Medicine of Case Western Reserve University, Cleveland, Ohio, USA

Contents

> Connective tissue diseases often prominently affect the skin, requiring dermatologists to play an important role in diagnosis and treatment of these patients. Herein we describe updates on the pathogenesis, clinical features, and treatment of 4 major connective tissue diseases: dermatomyositis, cutaneous lupus erythematosus, limited scleroderma (morphea), and cutaneous vasculitis. Many of these updates promise to improve clinical care of patients who suffer from dermatologic involvement of these diseases and are the result of research performed by dermatologists who have expertise in these conditions.

> Inflammatory granulomatous dermatitides include cutaneous sarcoidosis, necrobiosis lipoidica, granuloma annulare, and reactive granulomatous dermatitis. The etiopathogenesis of these disorders is not well understood; but the T helper 1 response mediated by interferon-gamma, tumor necrosis factor-alpha, and interleukin (IL) 1, 2, and 6 and the T helper 17 response mediated by IL-17 play a role. These inflammatory granulomatous disorders have extracutaneous manifestations, associations with systemic disease and medication triggers. The authors review these disorders, propose diagnostic and evaluative approaches to these diseases, and explore recent literature with regard to the etiopathogenesis and treatment of these entities.

> Comorbidities affecting dermatologic patients are of significant importance to providers and highly relevant for appropriate patient counseling, screening practices, prevention, and treatment. This article seeks to highlight several of the newest findings in the literature regarding comorbidities associated with dermatologic diseases including atopic dermatitis, hidradenitis suppurativa, alopecia areata, chronic urticaria, and the pemphigus family of immunobullous diseases. Further investigation is needed for associations between atopic dermatitis and pancreatic cancer and pemphigus family diseases and chronic obstructive pulmonary disease in order to better characterize the strength of these associations and clinical relevance.

> Skin cancer is reaching epidemic levels in the United States. Recent advances in the understanding of the pathophysiology of melanoma have allowed improved risk stratification in the revised American Joint Committee on Cancer (AJCC) criteria, new tests to capture patients at higher risk than their stage may indicate, and new treatments to offer hope and cures to patients with advanced disease.

> Immunosuppressed patients are at significantly increased risk of developing cutaneous malignancies. These malignancies are often more aggressive compared with the general population and require multidisciplinary care. This article highlights the incidence and risk factors of cutaneous malignancies in this cohort. The treatment and prevention strategies are discussed. There continues to be a need for

evidence-driven guidelines regarding the management of skin cancers in these patients.

Chikungunya and Zika virus infections are emerging diseases in the Americas, and dengue continues to be the most prevalent arthropod-borne virus in the world. These arbovirus diseases may spread by endemic transmission or as travel-related infections and have rapidly expanded their geographic distribution secondary to vector spread. All 3 share a similar clinical picture that includes a maculopapular rash. Zika is characterized by pruritic rash, low-grade fever, and arthralgia. Congenital nervous system malformations are a growing public-health concern. Chikungunya distinctive dermatologic manifestations include facial melanosis and bullous eruption. Dengue bleeding complications may be life-threatening and require inpatient management.

Cosmeceuticals are cosmetics that promise to deliver physiologically relevant benefits without the incorporation of prescription drugs. To entice consumers to purchase these premium priced products, a story must be told of how the cosmeceutical delivers on these appearance improvement promises. The backbone of any cosmeceutical skin care regimen is facial cleansing and moisturizing. This article reviews the novel ingredients and technologies used to achieve these benefits examining what is real and what is not.

Topical silicone gel is more beneficial than petrolatum-based products as an all-purpose wound dressing for granulating and sutured wounds, regardless of cause. Vaginal laser rejuvenation is effective in relieving genitourinary syndrome of menopause, stress urinary incontinence, vaginal relaxation syndrome, and related vulvar disorders. New cosmetic indications in the upper face for onabotulinumtoxinA have been approved by the Food and Drug Administration, whereas off-label treatments in the lower face increase in popularity. Clinical trials of uncomplexed daxibotulinumtoxinA demonstrate safety and efficacy lasting more than 6 months.

DERMATOLOGIC CLINICS

THE CLINICS ARE AVAILABLE ONLINE!
Access your subscription at:
www.theclinics.com

Preface
Hot Topics in Dermatology

This issue of *Dermatologic Clinics* offers a sizzling array of topics, which are all designated to be hot, topical, and clinically relevant to any practicing dermatologist or dermatology surgeon.

The theme is an offshoot of the American Academy of Dermatology (AAD) Hot Topics symposium, one of the most popular sessions at the annual meeting, which is a testament to both the theme and the faculty. I've had the honor of orchestrating the symposium several times, and I shall do so again at the annual meeting of AAD in Washington, DC in 2019. The symposium covers six to seven hot topics, as determined by members and registrants. This issue of *Dermatologic Clinics* addresses those topics and several others that were definitely warm, if not truly hot.

Some topics were obvious, such as acne, atopic dermatitis, psoriasis and biologic Rx, and melanoma. Others are perhaps less so, but they are still notable and important: connective tissue disease, co-morbidities, skin cancer/immunosuppression, contact dermatitis, granulomatous disease, new and emerging infectious diseases, and of course, cosmetics and cosmetic surgery.

I was fortunate to recruit a notable cadre of authors, all of whom are respected, seasoned experts in their fields, and several of whom covered the topics at the last annual AAD meeting. They are all good friends who accepted my invitation to join the writing adventure. The result is a rather striking and hopefully memorable issue. My thanks and compliments to all involved: the New Yorkers: Mark Lebwohl, Hilary Baldwin, and David Cohen; the Philadelphians: Nino Benedetto, and Misha Rosenbach; the Tar Heel, Zoe Draelos; the San Diegoan, Larry Eichenfield; the DC connection, Adam Friedman; the surgical Sooner: Tom Stasko; my Mexican amigo, Jose Dario Martinez; and my colleagues at the Clinic: Tony Fernandez and Alok Vij. Without them, individually and collectively, the issue would not have been possible. This was indeed a group effort, and the authors did the "heavy lifting." I was simply the maestro.

Last, my thanks to Bruce Thiers, for his invitation to oversee the issue and, Sara Watkins, the point person at Elsevier who helped me and the gang with editorial guidelines and direction. She helped to keep all of us "on track."

To you, the reader… sit back, turn the pages, and enjoy the final product.

Kenneth J. Tomecki, MD
Cleveland Clinic
9500 Euclid Avenue
Cleveland, OH 44195, USA

E-mail address:
TOMECKK@ccf.org

Dermatol Clin 37 (2019) ix
https://doi.org/10.1016/j.det.2018.09.001
0733-8635/19/© 2018 Published by Elsevier Inc.

Erratum

In the October 2018 issue of *Dermatologic Clinics* (Volume 36, Issue 4) devoted to Alternative Uses of Dermatoscopy, the authors' affiliations for the article "Dermoscopy of Lymphomas and Psuedolymphomas" were listed incorrectly. The correct affiliations are:

Caterina Bombonato, MD (a) Riccardo Pampena, MD (a), Aimillios Lallas, MD, MSc, PhD (b) Pellacani Giovanni, MD (c)*, Caterina Longo, MD, PhD (a, c)

a) Centro Oncologico ad Alta Tecnologia Diagnostica, Azienda Unità Sanitaria Locale – IRCCS di Reggio Emilia, Viale Risorgimento 80, Reggio Emilia 42123, Italy

b) First Department of Dermatology, Aristotle University, Hospital of Skin and Venereal Diseases, 124 Delfon Street, Thessaloniki 54643, Greece

c) Dermatology Department, University of Modena and Reggio Emilia, via del Pozzo 71, Modena 41124, Italy

Dermatol Clin 37 (2019) xi
https://doi.org/10.1016/j.det.2018.09.002
0733-8635/19/© 2018 Published by Elsevier Inc.

New Concepts, Concerns, and Creations in Acne

Justin W. Marson, BA[a], Hilary E. Baldwin, MD[b,c],*

KEYWORDS

- Acne • Acne scarring • Microbiome • Creatine kinase • Acne pipeline
- Gamma glutamyltransferase

KEY POINTS

- Creatine kinase should be monitored in athletic males on isotretinoin.
- Gamma glutamyltransferase is superior to other liver transaminases when following hepatic function of isotretinoin.
- Acne scarring is partly a result of delayed and inadequate treatment.
- The acne pipeline is rich with new chemical entities and combinations.
- Laser and light therapies for acne, while effective, need additional evidence-based data to support their use as a first-line therapy.

INTRODUCTION

Acne vulgaris is the most common condition treated by dermatologists worldwide. The literature is replete with new concepts regarding pathophysiology and therapeutic approaches, new concerns regarding appropriate therapeutic goals and the safety of laboratory monitoring, and the creation of new medications for the acne toolbox. The authors have chosen 5 topics that have new information to help physicians safely and effectively care for patients with acne.

WHICH TESTS ARE NECESSARY FOR PATIENTS ON ORAL ISOTRETINOIN?

Creatine Kinase

There have been many case series demonstrating correlations between oral isotretinoin (OI) and elevated creatine kinase (CK).[1–10] Webster and colleagues[1] found 44% of patients had at least 1 elevated CK on OI. Although females had similar frequency of 1-time elevated CK as males (22–30), males had over tenfold greater instances of multiple elevated CK on OI (57–1).[1] It is still unclear whether OI alone can elevate CK, or if synergy with a concurrent second offender (eg, exercise) elevates CK. There is currently neither consensus on the significance nor guidelines for management of elevated CK on OI, which is especially concerning, as there are multiple reports and at least 1 documented death from rhabdomyolysis (CK greater than 5 times normal value) on OI.[2–7]

Based on the current literature and their own experiences, the authors recommend baseline CK evaluation in all individuals prior to initiation of OI therapy (Table 1). Furthermore, the authors recommend regular monitoring of serum CK in male athletes who engage in strenuous physical activity and all individuals with abnormal serum CK at baseline. Monitoring may be titrated down after trending a patient's new baseline serum CK on OI and if he or she will not engage in supranormal physical activity while on OI or not exceed

Disclosure Statement: Mr J.W. Marson has no relevant disclosures. Dr H.E. Baldwin serves on the speaker's bureau for Galderma and Ortho Dermatologics, has or is conducting clinical trials for Dermira, Ortho Dermatologics, Novan, SolGel and Galderma, and is a medical advisor for BioPharmX.
[a] Rutgers Robert Wood Johnson Medical School, 675 Hoes Lane W, Piscataway, NJ 08854, USA; [b] The Acne Treatment and Research Center of the DermGroup, 310 Madison Avenue, Morristown, NJ 07960, USA; [c] Rutgers Robert Wood Johnson Medical Center, Piscataway, NJ 08820, USA
* Corresponding author. The Acne Treatment and Research Center of the DermGroup, 310 Madison Avenue, Morristown, NJ 07960.
E-mail address: hbaldwin@acnetrc.com

Dermatol Clin 37 (2019) 1–9
https://doi.org/10.1016/j.det.2018.07.002

Table 1
Authors' conclusion and recommendations regarding trending serum creatine kinase

Population	Baseline CK	Regular Activity	Unusually Intense Physical Activity	Recommendation
All	—	—	—	Baseline CK evaluation
All	Normal	None	None	One-time CK evaluation after reaching 0.5 mg/kg
All	Abnormal	None	None	Monthly CK evaluation
All	—	—	Yes	CK Evaluation 1–4 d after activity, especially in normally sedentary individuals
Male athletes	—	Yes	—	Monthly CK evaluation
Female athletes	—	Yes	—	Monthly CK evaluation, especially if baseline CK is (borderline) abnormal

5 times the reference of serum CK while on OI after engagement in supranormal strenuous physical activity. Patients who have serum CK elevations approaching or exceeding 5 times the normal laboratory values should discontinue or reduce either physical activity or OI dosage until their serum CK values return to average pre-OI therapy levels.

Liver Function

Liver function tests, traditionally alanine aminotransferase (ALT) and aspartate aminotransferase (AST), are often trended during OI therapy. However, these markers are also present in muscle tissue and even red blood cells.[1] In addition to the lack of tissue specificity, Webster found the meager rises in AST and ALT (highest values 191 and 118, respectively) correlated more with CK than with another liver marker, gamma-glutamyltransferase (GGT, highest value 102), suggesting elevated AST/ALT may originate from muscle not liver tissue. Altogether, GGT may be more specific for liver dysfunction during OI therapy.

IS THERE STRONG EVIDENCE FOR LIGHT/LASER THERAPY IN ACNE TREATMENT?

Laser/light-based therapies (LBT) use energy to excite endogenous (porphyrins) or exogenous photosensitive adjuncts and create radical oxygen species targeted either at *Propionibacterium acnes* or the sebaceous gland, reducing inflammation and sebum production.[11]

Barbaric and colleagues[11] compiled data about the efficacy of different LBTs and found that, by participant's global assessment of improvement, aminolevulinic acid photodynamic therapy (ALA-PDT) with blue light had no benefit over blue light alone, but 20% ALA-PDT with red light was more effective than 10% or 5% ALA-PDT (NNT of 6 and 4, respectively). They also found that methyl aminolevulinate (MAL-) PDT with red light was no better at reducing inflammatory or noninflammatory lesions than placebo cream and red light. The heterogeneous nature of the studies prevented Barbaric from finding high-quality evidence for the use of LBT for acne therapy.[11]

de Vries and colleagues[12] reported on the ability of LBTs to reduce acne lesions compared with either a control or baseline. They found moderate evidence for the use of single-pass IPL in reduction of both inflammatory and noninflammatory acne lesions compared with double pass and the use of diode laser in reduction of inflammatory lesions compared with no treatment. They also included studies comparing LBT with conventional therapies (blue light vs 1% clindamycin, blue light vs cumulative 54 mg/kg isotretinoin, IPL vs benzoyl peroxide, PDL vs 5% benzoyl peroxide gel) and found no significant differences between treatment groups, suggesting non-inferiority of LBT.

Many of the current studies were: underpowered (<100 participants), of insufficient duration (average 8 weeks), inadequately blinded, or did not have appropriate comparisons. Most findings compared different LBTs against each other or no therapy. Despite methodology hampering result quality, many of the studies reported significant reduction in acne lesions. As both de Vries and Barbaric have justly noted, more stringently designed studies are needed to determine the role of LBT as an adjunct or even monotherapy.

WHAT ROLE DOES THE CUTANEOUS MICROBIOME PLAY IN ACNE?
What Is the Microbiome, and What Is Its Role?

Skin is home to a vast collection of bacteria, viruses, and fungi termed the microbiome. Synergy among the various species cultivates commensal species while inhibiting pathogenic ones (eg, *Staphylococcus aureus*) through production of antimicrobial peptides (AMPs) and competition for resources.[13]

Studies now implicate changes in skin physiology and the microbiome in acne pathogenesis. Evidence suggests there is inherent epidermal barrier dysfunction in acne-prone skin, creating an inhospitable environment for commensal species.[13–15] Furthermore, acne regimens (eg, benzoyl peroxide, topical retinoids, OI) have been shown to further exacerbate the dysfunctional epidermal barrier, and, in the case of OI, even directly alter the microbiome after therapy.[16–21] This imbalance creates permissible conditions for pathologic strains of microbes implicated in infection and inflammation, such as virulent strains of *P acnes* (ie, *P acnes* IA1 phylotype) in the case of acne.[13,22–24]

Can Probiotics/Prebiotics Serve as Therapeutic Agents?

Studies suggests that probiotics (commensal species) and prebiotics, nonliving substances that promote beneficial bacteria, may have therapeutic potential against acne by mending the epidermal barrier.[22,23] Mottin and Suyenaga[25] investigated the use of probiotics and their AMPS and prebiotics in restoration of the microbiome and treatment of acne lesions.

Multiple in vitro studies have assessed the potential for targeted antimicrobial activity against *P acnes* (**Table 2**). Wang and colleagues[26] showed *Staphylococcus epidermidis,* especially when cultured with glycerol, interfered with the proliferation of *P acnes* obtained from the faces of healthy individuals. Oh and colleagues[27] found bacteriocin produced by *Lactococcus species HY 499* could inhibit growth of *P acnes* (and *Staphylococcus aureus, Staphylococcal epidermidis,* and *Streptococcus pyogenes*) without inducing type IV hypersensitivity. Studies have shown *Streptococcus salivarius,* isolated from the oro-/nasopharynx, produces a bacterocin-like inhibitory substance (BLIS) that inhibits proliferation of pathogenic

microbes (eg, group A *Streptococcus*) and certain strains of *P acnes* and downregulates genes moderated by NF-κB involved in innate immunity and interleukin (IL)-8 secretion and response.[28,29] In abdominal plastic skin explant models, Gueniche and colleagues[30] found that *Lactobacillus paracasei CNCM I-2116* was capable of mitigating substance P-induced tumor necrosis factor (TNF)-alpha release, vasodilation, edema, and mast cell granulation, and expediting barrier reconstruction simulated by decreased transepidermal water loss (TEWL).

Studies have also investigated clinical application of probiotics/prebiotics (**Table 3**). A double-blind, randomized control trial found 8 weeks of topical powdered fecal *Enterococcus faecalis SL-5* lotion (isolated from healthy adults) significantly reduced the number of pustules in individuals with mild-to-moderate acne compared with individuals with acne who were given vehicle.[31] Muizzuddin and colleagues[32] determined, after 4 days of daily spot-application of *Lactobacillus plantarum* extract solubilized in oil in water formula at 1% or 5%, the 5% solution had significant reduction in erythema and lesion size versus salicylate in 10 individuals. Kim and colleagues[33] found after 12 weeks of consuming fermented milk with 200 mg of lactoferrin, individuals with acne had a reduction in inflammatory lesions and sebum content—in total and lower triacylglycerol content—than individuals with acne who only consumed fermented milk.

Where Do We Stand Now with the Microbiome?

Although research is pursuing various species with promising anti-inflammatory and antimicrobial properties, there is no guarantee a single strain will work universally as an individual's microbiome is unique, dependent on genetics and their everyday environment. That being said, there is a need for more targeted therapies (as opposed to the systemic use of antibiotics and possible antibiotic resistance) with fewer adverse effects

Table 2
In vitro/ex vivo studies of probiotics/prebiotics as therapeutic agents

Study	Probiotic/Prebiotic	Active Compound/Mechanism of Action
Wang et al,[26] 2014	*Staphylococcus epidermidis*	Glycerol fermentation products
Oh et al,[27] 2006	*Lactococcus species HY 499*	Bacteriocin
Bowe et al,[28] 2006	*Streptococcus salivarius*	BLIS
Cosseau et al,[29] 2008	*Streptococcus salivarius*	BLIS
Gueniche et al,[30] 2010	*Lactobacillus paracasei CNCM I-2116*	Unidentified extract

Table 3
In vivo studies of probiotics/prebiotics as therapeutic agents

Study	Probiotic/ Prebiotic	Active Compound/ Mechanism of Action	Study Design	Vehicle	Control	Study Duration	# Patients
Kang et al,[31] 2009	*Enterococcus faecalis SL-5*	Enterocins (ESL5)	Double-blind randomized-controlled trial	Lotion	Vehicle	8 wk	70
Muizzuddin et al,[32] 2012	*Lactobacillus plantarum*	Unidentified AMP extract	CCT	Oil in water solution	1% Salicylate	4 d	10
Kim et al,[33] 2010	Lactoferrin	Lactoferrin	Double-blind randomized-controlled trial	Fermented milk	Fermented milk	12 wk	36

(most notable with oral isotretinoin) as adjuncts or possibly alternatives to acne therapy.

FACIAL ACNE SCARS: WHO GETS THEM, HOW CAN ONE REDUCE THE RISK, AND SHOULD THEY BE MANAGED?
Incidence

Strong epidemiologic data on the prevalence of acne scarring are lacking, and documentation of the severity of those scars is even less well described in the literature. In a large study conducted in Brazil, France, and the United States, 40% of current acne patients had some type of acne scarring.[34]

The importance of such statistics lies in not only the physical scars that may last a lifetime but, more importantly, the lifelong psychological scars that may affect patients' quality of life.[35] Scarring is an independent variable for suicide risk and depression.[36] Patients believe that scars impact their professional lives and reduce their future employability.[34] As it turns out, these patients are correct; they are being judged by others. In a digital online survey, Dreno and colleagues[37] demonstrated that subjects with facial acne scars are negatively perceived by society. The survey suggested that observers presumed a lack of good skin care habits and an overall neglect of health and hygiene on the part of the patients.

Who Gets Acne Scars?

Not everyone with acne develops scars. Furthermore, it is not always possible to predict who will scar or even which lesion is most likely to scar. Genetic factors likely predetermine the inflammatory response and ultimately the wound healing process resulting from the trauma of the acne lesion.[38]

Studies have shown that the magnitude and the type of inflammatory response are different in scar-formers versus nonformers, and that the process represents an altered wound healing response.[39–44]

Atrophic acne scars, often perceived as permanent and burnt out, are actually active and dynamic lesions. Lee and colleagues[43] showed the presence of inflammatory infiltrates in 77% of scars. Tan demonstrated that 34% of scars arose and subsequently resolved spontaneously during a 6-month observational study.[45] This implies that visible scars are not a done deal, and continued treatment beyond resolution of active acne lesions is warranted. The same study showed that the probability of an individual acne lesion producing a scar was 5.7%, highlighting the importance of early and aggressive acne therapy; every pimple is a sizable risk factor for scar.

Besides genetic predisposition, other factors have also been shown to contribute to the risk of facial acne scars (Table 4). Although acne of any severity, even mild, can result in scarring, more severe cases and highly inflamed lesions are more

Table 4
Acne products in clinical development

Class	Product
Antibacterial Agents	Minocycline gel Minocycline foam Sarecycline Nitric oxide gel
Retinoids	Trifarotene Tretinoin/BPO combination
Sebum inhibitors	Olumocostat glasaretil Cortexolone 17 α-propionate cream

likely to scar.[34,46,47] Acne relapse after initial successful therapy, increased body mass index (BMI), male gender, and a positive family history of severe acne have been associated with scar development.[45] One of the most consistent and significant factors associated with acne scar risk is delay in treatment.[34,46,47] The risk factors of acne severity and delay in treatment are both modifiable by early and aggressive treatment.

Treatment of Acne Scars

Treatment of acne scars is primarily non-pharmacologic. Fillers, laser, chemical and mechanical resurfacing techniques, microneedling, and surgical interventions (subcision and excisional techniques) have been shown to improve, but not normalize, the appearance of scars.[48–50] These treatments are not affordable by all, involve varying amounts of down time, and are not uniformly effective. Often the best-case scenario better—but not normal—ends in patient dissatisfaction.

Topical retinoids have been shown to improve fine lines and wrinkles in photoaged skin, presumably because of their ability to stimulate fibroblast production of procollagen.[51–54] Tretinoin, adapalene 0.3% gel, and adapalene 0.1%/BP2.5% have all been shown to reduce the development of acne scars and in some cases to improve the appearance of existing facial acne scars.[55–57] Most recently, adapalene 0.3%/BP2.5% gel was shown to prevent the formation and improve the appearance of existing facial acne scars in a 6-month, split-face, vehicle-controlled trial of moderate-severe active acne patients with scarring tendency.[58]

Taken together, all of the data point to an inevitable conclusion; treatment of facial acne scars is painful, expensive, time-consuming, and generally imperfect. Avoidance of scar formation is therefore of paramount importance. Many of the risk factors for scars, such as gender and family and genetic influences, are unmodifiable. Modifiable factors include early recognition of the scarring diathesis, early and aggressive treatment, and continued treatment well past the resolution of the last active acne lesion. Because not all acne scars are permanent, treatment geared to the both the resolution of active acne lesions and scars is warranted.

THE ACNE PIPELINE: WHAT DOES THE FUTURE HOLD?

The recent decade has marked an explosive increase in our knowledge of acne pathophysiology. Coincident with this is the recognition of the dire circumstance of worldwide antibiotic resistance and a call for dermatologists to be better stewards of the antibiotics that are used so readily for noninfectious conditions.[59,60] With this in mind, a more targeted approach to acne therapy, one less reliant on broad-spectrum antibiotics, has received full attention. New therapies that target the inflammatory cascade and sebum suppression, oral antibiotics with a narrower spectrum of activity, topical antibacterials with less risk of resistance and without systemic absorption, and probiotics are all in various stages of clinical development (**Table 5**).

ANTIMICROBIALS

Although the overall goal is to avoid the use of antimicrobials in the treatment of acne, they are undeniably useful. Clinicians are aware that there are patients in whom other therapies are ineffective or, for various reasons, unavailable for use. Because of decades of use, antibiotic resistance has become common, necessitating the development of new agents.[61–63]

Topical Agents

Minocycline
Minocycline, taken orally, is a highly effective medication for the treatment of acne. However, its delivery through the skin has been a challenge.

Minocycline gel is entering phase 3 trials. It has been shown in vivo to penetrate into the sebaceous glands and to produce no detectable levels in the systemic circulation.[64] In the phase 2b trial (N = 210), the 2% gel was found to produce a 25%, 43.3%, and 58.5% reduction in inflammatory lesions at 2, 4, and 12 weeks, respectively.[65] The investigator global assessment (IGA) showed a positive trend over the duration of the study. It was well tolerated with no photosensitivity or staining/bleaching of fabric noted.

Minocycline foam has completed its phase 3 trials with a 4% formulation. There was a statistically significant reduction in inflammatory and noninflammatory lesions.[66] One of the 2 studies, however, missed the IGA end point, and an additional, larger phase 3 trial is ongoing. The

Table 5 Risk factors for acne scarring	
	Risk Factors
Nonmodifiable	Genetic preponderance Male gender Family history of severe acne
Modifiable	Acne severity Disease relapse Increased BMI Delay in effective treatment

product was well tolerated and showed no systemic absorption.

Topical nitric oxide gel

Nitric oxide is a naturally occurring substance in the human body that has broad antimicrobial and anti-inflammatory properties. In phase 2 trials, the gel was shown to have significant efficacy against inflammatory and noninflammatory lesions, was well tolerated, and showed no systemic absorption.[67] In the phase 3 trial, there was a 50.3% and 42.4% reduction in inflammatory and noninflammatory lesions at week 12 (*P*<.001).[68] However only one1 of the 2 studies reached statistical significance with the IGA. Another phase 3 trial is underway.

Oral Agents

Sarecycline

Sarecycline is a tetracycline class antibiotic with a narrow spectrum of activity targeting *P acnes* and *Staphylococcus aureus* and more limited activity against gram-negative gastrointestinal organisms than minocycline and doxycycline.[69] It has also shown anti-inflammatory activity and has a long half-life enabling once-daily dosing. Combined, these features suggest that sarecycline may have improved efficacy and fewer adverse effects than current oral tetracyclines. In the phase 3 trials, efficacy endpoints—IGA success and mean percent reduction of inflammatory lesions from baseline—were both met with *P*<.0001.[70] There was a 50.4% reduction in inflammatory lesions but no statistically significant change in noninflammatory lesions. Adverse effects were limited and in keeping with other tetracyclines.

Retinoids

Trifarotene

Trifarotene is the first fourth-generation retinoid to be studied for acne vulgaris. It is a highly selective retinoic acid receptor-gamma (RAR-γ) agonist, which could potentially increase efficacy and/or decrease irritation compared with the less selective agents.[71] In a mouse model it was shown to reduce comedones and increase epidermal thickness in a dose-dependent manner, more effectively than either tretinoin 0.05% or tazarotene 0.1%.[71] The phase 3 trial was completed in November 2017, and results are pending.

Tretinoin/benzoyl peroxide combination

In the past, the challenge of this combination hinged on stabilizing tretinoin in the presence of benzoyl peroxide. In this product, the benzoyl peroxide and tretinoin are individually encapsulated in a silica core-shell structure, which has been shown to preserve the stability of the tretinoin. In a phase 2 trial, success in IGA and change in inflammatory and noninflammatory lesion counts were statistically significant compared with vehicle (*P*<.001 for all).[72] Phase 3 study is currently enrolling.

Sebum Production Inhibitors

Excessive and/or atypical sebaceous gland activity undeniably contributes to the pathogenesis of acne, and as such, numerous agents have been evaluated in the past with limited success.

Olumacostat glasaretil

Olumacostat glasaretil inhibits acetyl coenzyme A carboxylase, which is an enzyme responsible for fatty acid synthesis.[73] In phase 2 studies, its twice-daily use produced statistically significant reduction in inflammatory and noninflammatory lesions.[73] In a recent phase 3 study, however, the drug failed to meet its clinical end points, and its development in acne may be discontinued.

Cortexalone 17 α-propionate 1% cream

Cortexalone 17 α-propionate 1% cream is a topical peripherally selective steroidal antiandrogen with some anti-inflammatory properties. It has been shown to easily penetrate human skin, where it is metabolized into cortexolone, which lacks androgenic effects.[74] In the phase 2b study of 363 patients, all end points (IGA and inflammatory and noninflammatory lesions) were reached.[74] The phase 3 trial is currently underway.

REFERENCES

1. Webster GF, Webster TG, Grimes LR. Laboratory tests in patients treated with isotretinoin: occurrence of liver and muscle abnormalities and failure of AST and ALT to predict liver abnormality. Dermatol Online J 2017;23(5) [pii:13030/qt7rv7j80p].
2. Chen D, Rofsky HE. Reply. J Am Acad Dermatol 1985;12(3):583–5.
3. Heudes AM, Laroche L. Muscular damage during isotretinoin treatment. Ann Dermatol Venereol 1998; 125(2):94–7 [in French].
4. Landau M, Mesterman R, Ophir J, et al. Clinical significance of markedly elevated serum creatine kinase levels in patients with acne on isotretinoin. Acta Derm Venereol 2001;81(5):350–2.
5. McBurney EI, Rosen DA. Elevated creatine phosphokinase with isotretinoin. J Am Acad Dermatol 1984;10(3):528–9.
6. Kaymak Y. Creatine phosphokinase values during isotretinoin treatment for acne. Int J Dermatol 2008; 47(4):398–401.
7. McBurney EI, Rosen DA. Reply. J Am Acad Dermatol 1985;12(3):582–3.

8. Tillman DM, White SI, Aitchison TC. Isotretinoin, creatine kinase and exercise. Br J Dermatol 1990; 123(s37):22–3.

9. Lipinski JT, Schwimmer B. Elevated CPK and isotretinoin. J Am Acad Dermatol 1985;12(3):581–5.

10. Hartung B, Merk HF, Huckenbeck W, et al. Severe generalised rhabdomyolysis with fatal outcome associated with isotretinoin. Int J Legal Med 2012;126(6): 953–6.

11. Barbaric J, Abbott R, Posadzki P, et al. Light therapies for acne. Cochrane Database Syst Rev 2016;(9):CD007917.

12. de Vries FMC, Meulendijks AM, Driessen RJB, et al. The efficacy and safety of non-pharmacological therapies for the treatment of acne vulgaris: a systematic review and best-evidence synthesis. J Eur Acad Dermatol Venereol 2018;32(7):1195–203.

13. Byrd AL, Belkaid Y, Segre JA. The human skin microbiome. Nat Rev Microbiol 2018;16(3):143–55.

14. Yamamoto A, Takenouchi K, Ito M. Impaired water barrier function in acne vulgaris. Arch Dermatol Res 1995;287(2):214–8.

15. Meyer K, Pappas A, Dunn K, et al. Evaluation of seasonal changes in facial skin with and without acne. J Drugs Dermatol 2015;14(6):593–601.

16. Draelos ZD, Ertel KD, Berge CA. Facilitating facial retinization through barrier improvement. Cutis 2006;78(4):275–81.

17. Weber SU, Thiele JJ, Han N, et al. Topical alpha-tocotrienol supplementation inhibits lipid peroxidation but fails to mitigate increased transepidermal water loss after benzoyl peroxide treatment of human skin. Free Radic Biol Med 2003;34(2):170–6.

18. Herane MI, Fuenzalida H, Zegpi E, et al. Specific gel-cream as adjuvant to oral isotretinoin improved hydration and prevented TEWL increase–a double-blind, randomized, placebo-controlled study. J Cosmet Dermatol 2009;8(3):181–5.

19. Stucker M, Hoffmann M, Altmeyer P. Instrumental evaluation of retinoid-induced skin irritation. Skin Res Technol 2002;8(2):133–40.

20. Tagami H, Tadaki T, Obata M, et al. Functional assessment of the stratum corneum under the influence of oral aromatic retinoid (etretinate) in guinea-pigs and humans. Comparison with topical retinoic acid treatment. Br J Dermatol 1992;127(5):470–5.

21. Ryan-Kewley AE, Williams DR, Hepburn N, et al. Non-antibiotic isotretinoin treatment differentially controls Propionibacterium acnes on skin of acne patients. Front Microbiol 2017;8:1381.

22. Rocha MA, Bagatin E. Skin barrier and microbiome in acne. Arch Dermatol Res 2018;310(3):181–5.

23. Baldwin HE, Bhatia ND, Friedman A, et al. The role of cutaneous microbiota harmony in maintaining a functional skin barrier. J Drugs Dermatol 2017;16(1):12–8.

24. Dagnelie MA, Corvec S, Saint-Jean M, et al. Decrease in diversity of Propionibacterium acnes phylotypes in patients with severe acne on the back. Acta Derm Venereol 2018;98(2):262–7.

25. Mottin VHM, Suyenaga ES. An approach on the potential use of probiotics in the treatment of skin conditions: acne and atopic dermatitis. Int J Dermatol 2018. [Epub ahead of print].

26. Wang Y, Kuo S, Shu M, et al. Staphylococcus epidermidis in the human skin microbiome mediates fermentation to inhibit the growth of Propionibacterium acnes: implications of probiotics in acne vulgaris. Appl Microbiol Biotechnol 2014;98(1): 411–24.

27. Oh S, Kim SH, Ko Y, et al. Effect of bacteriocin produced by Lactococcus sp. HY 449 on skin-inflammatory bacteria. Food Chem Toxicol 2006; 44(8):1184–90.

28. Bowe WP, Filip JC, DiRienzo JM, et al. Inhibition of Propionibacterium acnes by bacteriocin-like inhibitory substances (BLIS) produced by Streptococcus salivarius. J Drugs Dermatol 2006;5(9):868–70.

29. Cosseau C, Devine DA, Dullaghan E, et al. The commensal Streptococcus salivarius K12 downregulates the innate immune responses of human epithelial cells and promotes host-microbe homeostasis. Infect Immun 2008;76(9):4163–75.

30. Gueniche A, Benyacoub J, Philippe D, et al. Lactobacillus paracasei CNCM I-2116 (ST11) inhibits substance P-induced skin inflammation and accelerates skin barrier function recovery in vitro. Eur J Dermatol 2010;20(6):731–7.

31. Kang BS, Seo JG, Lee GS, et al. Antimicrobial activity of enterocins from Enterococcus faecalis SL-5 against Propionibacterium acnes, the causative agent in acne vulgaris, and its therapeutic effect. J Microbiol 2009;47(1):101–9.

32. Muizzuddin N, Maher W, Sullivan M, et al. Physiological effect of a probiotic on skin. J Cosmet Sci 2012; 63(6):385–95.

33. Kim J, Ko Y, Park YK, et al. Dietary effect of lactoferrin-enriched fermented milk on skin surface lipid and clinical improvement of acne vulgaris. Nutrition 2010;26(9):902–9.

34. Dreno B, Layton A, Bettoli V, et al, on behalf of the Global Alliance to Improve Outcomes in Acne. Evaluation of the prevalence, risk factors, clinical characteristics, and burden of acne scars among active acne patients who have consulted a dermatologist in Brazil, France and the US. Presented at: 23rd EADV Congress. Amsterdam, The Netherlands, October 8–12, 2014:PO24.

35. Layton A, Seukeran D, Cunliffe W. Scarred for life? Dermatology 1997;195(Suppl 1):15–24.

36. Cotterill J, Cunliffe W. Suicide in dermatological patients. Br J Dermatol 1997;137:246–50.

37. Dreno B, Tan J, Kang S, et al. How people with facial acne scars are perceived in society: an online survey. Dermatol Ther (Heidelb) 2016;6(2):207–18.

38. English R, Shenefelt P. Keloids and hypertrophic scars. Dermatol Surg 1999;25(8):631–8.
39. Thiboutot D, Gollnick H, Bettoli V, et al. New insights into the management of acne: an update from the global alliance to improve outcomes in acne group. J Am Acad Dermatol 2009;60(Suppl 5):S1–50.
40. Goodman G. Management of post-acne scarring. What are the options for treatment? Am J Clin Dermatol 2000;1:3–17.
41. Holland D, Jeremy A, Roberts S, et al. Inflammation in acne scarring: a comparison of the responses in lesions from patients prone and not prone to scar. Br J Dermatol 2004;150:72–81.
42. Kang S, Cho S, Chung J, et al. Inflammation and extracellular matrix degradation mediated by activated transcription factors nuclear factor-kappaB and activator protein-1 in inflammatory acne lesions in vivo. Am J Pathol 2005;166:1691–9.
43. Lee W, Jung H, Lim H, et al. Serial sections of atrophic acne scars help in the interpretation of microscopic findings and the selection of good therapeutic modalities. J Eur Acad Dermatol Venereol 2013;27:643–6.
44. Saint-Jean M, Khammari A, Jasson F, et al. Different cutaneous innate immunity profiles in acne patients with and without atrophic scars. Eur J Dermatol 2016;26:68–74.
45. Tan J, Bourdes V, Bissonette R, et al. Prospective study of pathogenesis of atrophic acne scars and role of macular erythema. J Drugs Dermatol 2017;16(6):566–73.
46. Layton A, Henderson C, Cunliffe W. A clinical evaluation of acne scarring and its incidence. Clin Exp Dermatol 1994;19:303–8.
47. Tan J, Tang J, Fung K, et al. Development and validation of a scale for acne scar severity (SCAR-S) of the face and trunk. J Cutan Med Surg 2010;14:156–60.
48. Jacob C, Dover J, Kaminer M. Acne scarring: a classification system and review of treatment options. J Am Acad Dermatol 2001;45:109–17.
49. Goodman G. Postacne scarring: a review of its pathophysiology and treatment. Dermatol Surg 2000;26:857–71.
50. Jemec G, Jemec B. Acne: treatment of scars. Clin Dermatol 2004;22:434–8.
51. Fisher G, Datta S, Wang Z, et al. c-Jun-dependent inhibition of cutaneous procollagen transcription following ultraviolet irradiation is revered by all-trans retinoic acid. J Clin Invest 2000;106:663–70.
52. Kang S, Fisher G, Voorhees J. Photoaging and topical tretinoin: therapy, pathogenesis and prevention. Arch Dermatol 1997;133:1280–4.
53. Cho S, Lowe L, Hamilton T, et al. Long-term treatment of photoaged human skin with topical retinoic acid improves epidermal cell atypia and thickens the collagen band in papillary dermis. J Am Acad Dermatol 2005;53:769–74.
54. Griffiths C, Russman A, Majmudar G, et al. Restoration of collagen formation in photodamaged human skin by tretinoin (retinoic acid). N Engl J Med 1993;329:530–5.
55. Losson M, Leung S, Chien A, et al. Adapalene 0.3% gel shows efficacy for the treatment of atrophic acne scars. Dermatol Ther (Heidelb) 2018;8(2):245–57.
56. Harris D, Buckley C, Ostlere L. Topical retinoic acid in the treatment of fine acne scarring. Br J Dermatol 1991;125(1):81–2.
57. Dreno B, Tan J, Rlvier M, et al. Adapalene 0.1%/BP 2.5% gel reduces the risk of atrophic scar formation in moderate inflammatory acne: a split face randomized controlled trial. J Eur Acad Dermatol Venereol 2017;31(4):737–42.
58. Dreno B, Bissonnette R, Gagne-Henley A, et al. Prevention and reduction of atrophic acnes cars with adapalene 0.3%/BP 2.5% gel in subjects with moderate or severe facial acne. Results of a 6-month randomized, vehicle-controlled trial using intra-individual comparison. Am J Clin Dermatol 2018;19(2):275–86.
59. Sinnott S, Bhate K, Margolis D. Antibiotics and acne: an emerging iceberg of antibiotic resistance? Br J Dermatol 2016;174(6):1127–8.
60. Del Rosso J, Webster G, Rosen T, et al. Status report from the scientific panel on antibiotic use in dermatology of the American Acne and Rosacea Society. J Clin Aesthet Dermatol 2016;9(4):18–24.
61. Fan Y, Hao F, Wang W, et al. Multicenter cross-sectional observational study of antibiotic resistance and the genotypes of Propionibacterium acnes isolated from Chinese patients with acne vulgaris. J Dermato 2016;43(4):406–13.
62. Mendoza N, Hernandez P, Tyring S. Antimicrobial susceptibility of Propionibacterium acnes isolates from acne patients in Columbia. Int J Dermatol 2013;52(6):688–92.
63. Schafer F, Fich F, Lam M, et al. Antimicrobial susceptibility and genetic characteristics of Propionibacterium acnes isolated from patients with ace. Int J Dermatol 2013;52(4):418–25.
64. Nagavarapu U. Development and assessment of BPX-01, a novel topical minocycline gel for treatment of acne vulgaris. Presented at: American Academy of Dermatology Annual Meeting. Orlando, Florida, March 3–7, 2017.
65. Alexis A, Del Rosso J, Desai S, et al. Rapid improvement with BPX-01 minocycline topical gel in the treatment of moderate-severe inflammatory acne vulgaris. Poster Fall Clinical Dermatology Conference. Las Vegas, Nevada, September 18, 2017.
66. Gold S, et al. The efficacy and safety of FMX101, minocycline foam 4% for the treatment of acne

vulgaris. Poster Winter Clinical Dermatology Conference. Kauai, Hawaii, January, Jan 12-18, 2018.

67. Baldwin H, Blanco D, McKeever C, et al. Results of a phase 2 efficacy and safety study with SB204, an investigational topical nitric oxide-releasing drug for the treatment of acne vulgaris. J Clin Aesthet Dermatol 2016;9(8):12–8.

68. Hebert A. Evaluation of the efficacy, safety and tolerability of SB204 4% once daily in subjects with moderate-severe acne vulgaris treated topically for up to 52 weeks. Poster American Academy of Dermatology annual meeting. San Diego, Calfornia, February 1-6, 2018.

69. Leyden J, Sniukiene M, Berk D, et al. Efficacy and safety of oral sarecycline for the treatment of moderate to severe facial acne vulgaris. Presented at the 75th annual meeting of the American Academy of Dermatology. Orlando, Florida, March 3–7, 2017.

70. Kircik L, Bhatia N, Lain E, et al. Once-Daily Oral Sarecycline 1.5 mg/kg/day for moderate to severe acne vulgaris. Poster annual meeting of the American Academy of Dermatology. San Diego, California, February 1-6, 2018.

71. Thoreau E, Arlabosse J, Bouix-Peter C, et al. Structure-based design of Trifarotene (CD5789), a potent and selective RARγ agonist for the treatment of acne. Bioorg Med Chem Lett 2018;28(10):1736–41.

72. Available at: www.Solgel.gsc-web.com/events-and-presentations. Accessed February 14, 2018.

73. Bissonnette R, Poulin Y, Drew J, et al. Olumacostat glasaretil, a novel topical sebum inhibitor, in the treatment of acne vulgaris: a phase IIa, multicenter randomized, vehicle-controlled study. J Am Acad Dermatol 2017;76(1):33–9.

74. Available at: www.cassiopea.com. Accessed June 20, 2018.

Atopic Dermatitis
New Developments

Ayan Kusari, MA[a,b,c], Allison M. Han, BA[a,b,c], David Schairer, MD[a,b,c],
Lawrence F. Eichenfield, MD[a,b,c],*

KEYWORDS

- Atopic dermatitis • Eczema • Pathogenesis • Treatment • Comorbidities • Prevention

KEY POINTS

- New insights into the genetic and environmental underpinnings of atopic dermatitis confirm the role of barrier dysfunction and immune activation in this chronic, inflammatory disease.
- Barrier protein deficiency may play a greater role in non-white populations than previously thought.
- The natural history of atopic dermatitis is far less uniform than previously believed.
- Across multiple independent cohorts, a significant minority of patients have disease that persists beyond the onset of adolescence.
- Several promising topical and oral therapies have recently become available to patients, and many more are currently being developed. These therapies target various sites and pathways within the immune system, including phosphodiesterase 4, JAK-STAT, aryl hydrocarbon receptor and T-helper 2 cytokines.

INTRODUCTION

The 2010s have been called the decade of eczema, and for good reason. Exciting developments in basic science are reshaping our fundamental understanding of atopic dermatitis (AD). Research has expanded our knowledge of the epidemiology of AD, showing subsets of the population with varying timing of onset and disease course, and the spectrum of comorbidities is being better understood. The treatment arsenal is broadening, with multiple new topical and systemic agents being approved and many under investigation. Herein, we aim to provide a comprehensive picture of these recent developments in our understanding of AD pathogenesis, epidemiology as well as preventative measures and treatment.

PATHOGENESIS
Barrier Dysfunction and Immune Abnormalities

Both dysfunction of the epidermal barrier and immune dysregulation are known to play a role in the pathogenesis of AD. The question of which

Disclosure Statement: Mr A. Kusari, Ms A.M. Han, and Dr L.F. Eichenfield all consent to publication of this article in its current form. Mr A. Kusari and Ms A.M. Han report no conflicts of interest or financial disclosures related to this case. Dr L.F. Eichenfield reports no financial relationships relevant to the article. Dr L.F. Eichenfield has been a principal investigator for, Galderma Laboratories, LP, Medimetriks, and Ortho Dermatology and he has received compensation for his work as a consultant for Anacor/Pfizer, Dermavant, Dermira, Leo, Lilly, Novan, Novartis, Regeneron/Sanofi and Ortho Dermatology. This project was partially supported by the National Institutes of Health, Grant TL1TR001443 CTSA funding, and the Rady Children's Hospital/UCSD Eczema and Inflammatory Skin Disease Center.

[a] Division of Pediatric and Adolescent Dermatology, Rady Children's Hospital, 8010 Frost Street, Suite 602, San Diego, CA 92123, USA; [b] Department of Dermatology, University of California, San Diego School of Medicine, 9500 Gilman Drive, La Jolla, CA 92093, USA; [c] Department of Pediatrics, University of California, San Diego School of Medicine, 9500 Gilman Drive, La Jolla, CA 92093, USA
* Corresponding author. Division of Pediatric and Adolescent Dermatology, Rady Children's Hospital, 8010 Frost Street, Suite 602, San Diego, CA 92123, USA.
E-mail address: leichenfield@rchsd.org

Dermatol Clin 37 (2019) 11–20
https://doi.org/10.1016/j.det.2018.07.003
0733-8635/19/© 2018 Elsevier Inc. All rights reserved.

comes first may be debated, but it is clear that both genetic and environmental factors influence both, and that both contribute to AD development and disease expression.[1] Dry skin is a hallmark of AD; lesional and nonlesional skin of patients with AD contain decreased barrier-stabilizing proteins and lipids. Keratinocytes in the stratum corneum lose their cell membranes, replaced by a layer of ceramides, cholesterol, and fatty acids, and surrounding this is a layer that develops a cornified envelope rich in loricrin, involucrin, and small proline-rich particles. Loricrin, along with the structural protein filaggrin, is downregulated in the face of inflammation, as shown in a study of cells exposed to cytokines tumor necrosis factor-alpha and IL-4.[2] IL-4, along with IL-13, IL-22, IL-31, thymic stromal-derived lymphopoietin, and others have been shown to be dysregulated in AD.[3] Many, particularly IL-4 and IL-13, are related to the activation or activity of T-helper type 2 (Th2) cells, and also seem to inhibit terminal differentiation of keratinocytes.[4]

Transepidermal Water Loss in Atopic Dermatitis

As a consequence of skin barrier compromise in patients with AD, transepidermal water loss (TEWL) is increased compared with individuals without disease. High TEWL in early infancy has been associated with later development of AD in several studies. A study of 1903 Irish neonates showed that arm TEWL greater than 9.0 g/m^2/h on the second day of life significantly predicted later development of AD.[5] A Japanese group, performing a similar study, measured TEWL from the forehead within the first 7 days of life and found that a forehead TEWL cutoff of 6.5 g/m^2/h was optimal for predicting later development of AD.[6] One study involving 116 children in Norway found a strong correlation between high TEWL at 6 months in infants without a clinical diagnosis of AD and the subsequent development of AD by 24 months.[7] Those with a TEWL of greater than 6.5 were at increased risk of developing AD later in life. A recent Korean study also seems to support a relationship between high early TEWL and later development of AD.[8] These observations have rationalized an approach to use early moisturizers to attempt to prevent AD.

Genetics

New insights into the genetic underpinnings of AD confirm the significant role played by barrier protein mutations and point toward an association between such mutations and persistent disease. Previously, the heritability of AD has been established in twin studies, with a pairwise concordance rate of 0.72 among identical twins in a large Danish study.[9] By far, mutations in the FLG gene, which encodes filaggrin, remain the most commonly identified genetic risk factor for the development of AD. When there is discordance between fraternal twins or siblings, differential inheritance of filaggrin mutations are most commonly responsible. In Northern Europeans, the R501X, 2282del4, and R2447X loss-of-function mutations in FLG seem to account for the majority of genetic discrepancy between such sibling pairs.[10] Estimates of FLG mutation prevalence among European patients with moderate or severe AD are as high as 50%.[11] In a recent cohort of 60 African American patients, FLG2 (rather than FLG) mutations were significantly associated with more persistent AD.[12] This finding is of note, because previous studies had not consistently shown a role for FLG mutations in mutations for African Americans with AD.[13,14] FLG2, like FLG, is located within the epidermal differentiation complex on chromosome 1q21, but had not previously been implicated in AD.

Despite the plethora of genes linked to AD, cases of AD strongly associated with a single gene mutation are rare. Recently, germline mutations in the CARD11 gene, which encodes a membrane-associated guanylyl kinase involved in lymphocyte signaling, was identified as a potential single-gene cause of AD in 8 patients from 4 families.[15] T lymphocytes extracted from these patients exhibited deficient mTORC1 and interferon-γ signaling, but supplementation with glutamine seemed to partially correct the lymphocyte dysfunction. If CARD11 signaling is found to play a role in AD pathogenesis outside the context of familial mutations, then glutamine supplementation may perhaps be an effective adjunctive therapy for some patients with AD.

Microbiome

The human skin microbiome is dominated by 4 phyla of bacteria—Firmicutes, Proteobacteria, Bacteroidetes, and Actinobacteria.[16] Increased gastrointestinal colonization with Staphylococcus and Streptococcus, which are members of the phylum Firmicutes, has been associated with obesity[17] (leading to headlines such as "4 Ways to Get Firm and Cute by Lowering Firmicutes"[18]). In AD, however, the picture is more complex. Staphylococcus aureus species density is increased in AD lesional skin, as are the commensal coagulase-negative staphylococcus species Staphylococcus epidermidis and Staphylococcus hominis.[16] However, S epidermidis species density is not increased to the same extent as *S aureus* and both *S epidermidis* and *S hominis* are known to have significant antimicrobial activity against *S aureus*. *S epidermidis* produces bacteriocidins that exhibit anti-*S aureus* activity; its serine protease Esp inhibits *S aureus* biofilm formation, whereas its phenol-soluble modulins decrease *S aureus* growth.[19] Esp, in particular, selectively degrades human fibronectin and fibrinogen, which are key receptor proteins that mediate *S aureus* biofilm formation, and acts in synergy with human antimicrobial peptides such as LL-37.[19] The application of antimicrobial peptides from coagulase-negative *Staphylococcus*, as well as direct application of coagulase-negative *Staphylococcus* strains, to the skin of humans with AD has recently been shown to decrease *S aureus* colonization and are being studied in patients with AD, and preclinical studies using *Roseomonas mucosa* application for AD have been performed.[20,21]

Effect of Environment

Environmental factors, including tobacco smoke, atmospheric humidity, and temperature, are known to play an important role in the development of AD. Environmental tobacco smoke, in particular, nearly doubles the risk of AD development.[22] A study of 1669 toddlers found that elevated urine levels of cotinine, a metabolite of nicotine, predicted later development of AD.[22]

Fluctuations in air temperature and humidity are commonly reported as AD triggers. Dry air is commonly believed to promote AD flares. This finding is supported by recent analysis of the National Survey of Children's Health data, a representative sample of 91,642 US children under the age of 18. A multivariate analysis controlling for age, sex, race, and household income found that children living in areas with environmental humidity in the highest quartile were the least likely to develop eczema. This analysis also showed that children exposed to more UV light seem to be relatively protected from eczema as well. These findings are not surprising, given that moisturization is an integral part of AD care, and narrowband UV phototherapy is an effective treatment for AD.[23]

However, heat and humidity are not uniformly associated with reduced symptom severity. Heat and humidity may promote sweating and sweat irritates the skin. A study of 25 children with AD found that hot, damp weather and self-reported sweating all predicted disease flare.[24]

CLINICAL PRESENTATION

AD was traditionally regarded as a disease with a fairly consistent natural history, characterized by onset in early childhood and remission in most patients by adolescence. However, new research identifying subgroups within the AD population has challenged this notion.[25]

In an analysis of 2 birth cohorts totaling 13,546 subjects from the Netherlands and the United Kingtom, 6 latent classes representing subphenotypes of AD were identified.[25] These groups were (1) early onset, early resolving, (2) early onset, late resolving, (3) early onset, persistent, (4) mid-onset, resolving, (5) late onset, resolving, and (6) transient or unaffected. Because the 6 groups were present, in remarkably similar proportions, across 2 unrelated cohorts in 2 countries, they were felt to represent genuine disease-related subgroups rather than artifact. In both cohorts, most patients (approximately 60%) were categorized as transient or unaffected. The second most common subphenotype of AD was early onset–early resolving, characterized by resolution in most patients by age 7. The other categories were less common, accounting for approximately 4% to 7% of patients with AD each, but in all, persistent or late resolving forms of AD accounted for a 10% to 14% of patients with AD. Females were more likely than males to be in the late onset or persistent categories and associations with asthma, parental history of atopic disease, and elevated IgE were stronger in the persistent categories.

PAIN, COMORBIDITIES, AND PREVENTATIVE MEASURES
Pain in Atopic Dermatitis

In 2016, Simpson and colleagues[26] explored AD symptomatology and showed that many patients with AD consider their AD painful. Using the EQ-5D, a general health quality-of-life questionnaire, the researchers asked patients about their AD symptoms and quality of life. They found that 76.8% of patients reported moderate or extreme pain with AD. In a 2017 survey of 305 adolescents and adults with AD, 144 patients (42.7%) reported skin pain and 42 patients (13.8%) reported severe or very severe pain.[27] Most respondents thought that skin pain was related to both itch and scratching.[27] These findings indicate that skin pain is an important finding in AD and may constitute a disease burden distinct from and compounding the burden of itch.

Atopy, Atopic Dermatitis, and Psychosocial Comorbidities

The atopic diathesis is well-studied and individuals with AD are more likely to have asthma,[28] food allergy,[29] contact dermatitis,[30] and allergic rhinitis.[31]

Numerous psychosocial comorbidities are also associated with AD. Perhaps the best-studied mental health comorbidity associated with AD is attention deficit hyperactivity disorder (ADHD). This finding is perhaps unsurprising, given the *Diagnostic and Statistical Manual of Mental Disorders*, 5th edition, diagnostic criteria for ADHD, which includes criteria such as "fidgeting" and "difficulty remaining seated," both of which may be observed in an itchy child. However, a clinical diagnosis of ADHD requires at least 12 symptoms—6 in the domain of inattentiveness and 6 in the domain of hyperactivity. Pruritus alone would be unlikely to explain 12 ADHD symptoms. Clinical ADHD seems to be more common in children with AD; a cross-sectional study of 92,642 children under the age of 18 found showed a 2-fold increase in ADHD risk with AD.[32,33] Pruritus in AD interferes with sleep and sleep is known to be important for neural development in children.[34]

Antihistamines, commonly used in AD care, have been associated with ADHD in patients with AD. Children taking antihistamines for AD seem to be at greater risk of developing ADHD symptoms than those who do not take antihistamines (odds ratio, 1.88).[35] More research is needed to uncover the mechanism for this effect, as well as its true extent.

In adolescence, AD is associated with elevated rates of anxiety disorders, particularly social anxiety disorder and general anxiety disorder.[36] This phenomenon may be due to self-consciousness related to physical appearance at this age. A recent study using the Dermatology Life Quality Index score showed that female gender and facial eczema are associated with particularly low quality of life.[37] AD is associated with increased risks of depression and suicidality; patients with more severe disease and females are at increased risk.[36] Elderly patients with AD are the age groups most likely to be depressed.[36] In adult patients with AD, estimates of anxiety or depression range from 10% to 22%,[26,38] with depressive symptoms present in as many as 43% to 46%.[26,38]

Metabolic Comorbidities in Atopic Dermatitis

AD has been associated with obesity in children[39] and adults[40]; however, current evidence is limited to retrospective case-control studies and causation may not be imputed. However, this association is biologically plausible given increased levels of proinflammatory cytokines seen in patients with AD.[40] By contrast, children with type 1 diabetes mellitus, a Th1-mediated disease, seem to be less likely to develop AD (a Th2-mediated disease) compared with well-matched controls.[41]

Measures to Prevent Atopic Dermatitis and Associated Comorbidities

Recently, early use of topical emollients has shown promise in the prevention of AD. In 2010, a study involving 22 neonates at high risk of AD development, defined as having 1 parent or sibling who currently or previously met the International Study on Asthma and Allergy in Childhood criteria for AD showed a significantly decreased rate of AD development (15%) compared with the expected 30% to 50% rate of AD development by 2 years.[42] Subsequently, a larger study involving 124 high-risk patients from the US and the UK was performed and showed that once-daily full-body emollient therapy starting within 3 weeks of birth decreased the relative risk of AD development at 6 months by 50%.[43] In the pilot study, Cetaphil cream (Galderma Laboratories, Fort Worth, TX), an oil-in-water, petrolatum-based cream was used.[42] In the larger study, a variety of creams and ointments were used in a nonrandom manner, including Cetaphil cream, Aquaphor ointment (Beiersdorf, Chester, OH), sunflower seed oil (William Hodgson and Co, Congleton, UK), Doublebase Gel (Dermal Laboratories, Hitchin, UK), and liquid paraffin 50% in white soft paraffin.

Peanut Allergy Prevention in Patients with Atopic Dermatitis

AD is a major risk factor for the development of peanut allergy, which is the food allergy with the highest rate of anaphylaxis and emergency care requirements. Early peanut introduction in patients with AD has been shown to reduce risk of peanut allergy, which is among the deadliest of food allergies and coincides with AD in many children.[44] Whereas the conventional wisdom was to delay introduction of high-risk foods in high-risk individuals, the results of the groundbreaking Learning Early About Peanut (LEAP) study indicate that children with severe eczema or egg allergy can benefit from moderate weekly peanut protein consumption. In the LEAP study, 640 infants aged 4 to 11 months with severe eczema or egg allergy were randomized to peanut avoidance until age 5 or consumption of 6 g of peanut protein per week. At the study's conclusion, the prevalence of peanut allergy in the avoidance group was 13.7%, whereas the prevalence of peanut allergy in the consumption group was 1.9% ($P<.001$).[45] The subsequent LEAP-On study, which extended the LEAP study by 12 months (months 60–72), showed that, even after 1 year of peanut avoidance, early exposure to peanuts in the first 60 months of life was protective against the development of peanut allergy (4.8% vs 18.6% peanut allergy prevalence).[46] Based on these results, an expert panel sponsored by the National Institute of Allergy and Infectious Diseases issued guidelines in 2017 recommending taking steps toward early introduction of peanuts in high-risk children, namely, those with severe eczema, egg allergy, or both. Per their recommendations, these high-risk children should undergo testing for peanut allergy with peanut-specific IgE or skin prick testing.[47] Those without evidence of peanut allergy on peanut-specific IgE or skin prick testing are recommended, under the new guidelines, to undergo early peanut introduction by 4 to 6 months of age. The National Institute of Allergy and Infectious Diseases panel also recommended introduction of peanut around 6 months in infants with mild-to-moderate eczema, and introduction in accordance with family preferences for patients without eczema or egg allergy.[47] The major practice implication of these guidelines is that all infants with severe AD should be evaluated with peanut peanut-specific IgE or skin prick testing, to guide early feeding of peanut protein and to prevent peanut allergy.

NEW TOPICAL THERAPIES
Crisaborole and Other Phosphodiesterase 4 Inhibitors

Phosphodiesterase (PDE) enzymes degrade cyclic nucleotides, including cyclic adenosine monophosphate and cyclic guanosine monophosphate. Different PDE enzymes are expressed in different cell types and have different functions. Many PDE enzymes are involved in atopic and inflammatory processes. Indeed, the first known PDE inhibitor may be caffeine; in 1859, an asthmatic London physician by the name of Henry Hyde Salter published a report of his own asthma improving after drinking 2 cups of strong coffee.[48] Caffeine has since been confirmed to have weak anti-PDE properties, as does the once widely used asthma medication theophylline.[49] PDE4 seems to be preferentially expressed in inflammatory cells, including those involved in chronic obstructive pulmonary disease, psoriasis, and AD. The PDE4 inhibitor apremilast has been approved by the US Food and Drug Administration (FDA) for use in psoriasis since 2014, whereas roflumilast has been FDA-approved for use in chronic obstructive pulmonary disease since 2011.[50] Oral PDE4 inhibitors have are less immune suppressing than oral corticosteroids, but are associated with significant nausea, vomiting, diarrhea, and abdominal pain at therapeutic doses. Given these systemic effects with oral administration, a topical option for skin disease was sought. Of the topical PDE4 inhibitors

studied in AD, crisaborole is the best-studied and the only one with FDA approval at this writing. Crisaborole was approved in December 2016 for the treatment of mild to moderate AD. Two large, multicenter studies, AD-301 and AD-302, involving a total of 1522 patients age 2 or older with AD showed a greater person of clear and almost clear scores in the treatment groups compared with vehicle control.[51] However, these trials were notable for their strong vehicle effect—with 40.6% in the vehicle control group achieving clear/almost clear with a 2 or more grade improvement in the AD-301 study,[51] leading to questions about the true efficacy of the active ingredient. The most common adverse effect of crisaborole seems to be stinging or burning at the application site. AD flare (owing to inadequate disease control) and application site infection were also reported in these trials. Absorption of the active compound seems to be limited, and gastrointestinal adverse effects are rare, reported in less than 2% of patients in the AD-301/302 studies. A 48-week, open-label extension involving 517 patients from the AD-301/302 studies, termed AD-303, did not analyze efficacy but confirmed the safety-related findings of the original studies.[52]

Aside from the 8 ongoing studies on crisaborole, there are multiple studies involving other topical PDE4 inhibitors for AD.[53,54]

Janus Kinase Inhibitors

In AD, Janus kinase/signal transducer and activator of transcription (JAK/STAT) signaling likely plays a major role. There are 4 major JAK proteins—JAK1, JAK2, JAK3, and tyrosine kinase 2. Differentiation of naive CD4 calls into Th2 cells depends on IL-4 cytokine production, which in turn depends on JAK1, JAK3, and STAT6 signaling.[55] JAK1 and JAK2 are also involved in antibody class switching to IgE in B cells. IL-6 and IL-23 signaling, which promotes CD4[+] T-cell differentiation into Th17, involves STAT3 downstream, and Th17 activity is known to play a role in acute AD. Human thymic stromal-derived lymphopoietin, which promotes CD4[+] T-cell differentiation into Th2, also involves JAK1, JAK2, STAT1, and STAT3 downstream. Thus, JAK/STAT signaling through multiple pathways (and multiple JAKs) seems to play a role in AD pathogenesis. This finding is in contrast with other diseases, such as psoriasis and alopecia areata, in which only 1 JAK pathway is predominantly involved.

Currently, several oral and intravenous JAK inhibitors are FDA approved for diseases other than AD. Tofacitinib is a JAK1/3 inhibitor approved for rheumatoid arthritis in patients who are unable to tolerate, or are refractory to, methotrexate. Ruxolitinib is a JAK1/2 inhibitor approved for high-risk myelofibrosis and polycythemia vera unresponsive to, or in patients unable to tolerate, hydroxyurea. One systemic JAK inhibitor is FDA approved to treat AD at present; however, this agent, oclacitinib, is only approved for AD in dogs.

The first trial of topical JAK inhibitors for AD was published in 2015, involving 69 adult patients with mild to moderate AD.[56] In this study, adults treated with 2% tofacitinib ointment showed 81.7% decrease in the Eczema Area and Severity Index (EASI) score at the end of 4 weeks of treatment, compared with a 29.9% mean decrease in the EASI score with the vehicle control group.[56] More recently, the topical ointment formulation of the investigational JAK inhibitor JTE-052 was shown to have a significantly improved modified EASI score at 4 weeks at multiple strengths compared with vehicle control, with the 3% strength of JTE-052 comparable with topical tacrolimus.[57,58] A phase II, multicenter study involving this agent has recently been completed. A trial comparing ruxolitinib phosphate cream (INC8018424) with triamcinolone 0.1% cream is currently ongoing, and pediatric trials of ruxolitinib and other topical JAK inhibitors are in process or in planning.

Tapinarof

Tapinarof is a novel agent that is believed to act by modulating the aryl hydrocarbon receptor. Topical tapinarof may be an effective treatment for AD. This study involved 247 patients aged 12 to 65 years who received 0.5% or 1.0% tapinarof cream, either daily or twice-daily. Of those receiving 1% tapinarof cream twice daily, 53% achieved the primary endpoint, IGA clear/almost clear and minimum 2-grade improvement by week 12, compared with 34% of those receiving 0.5% tapinarof cream daily, and 24% to 28% of those in the vehicle control groups. These findings indicate that tapinarof cream is a promising treatment for AD in adolescent and adult patients.[59]

Bleach Baths

Bleach (sodium hypochlorite solution) has been used as a disinfectant for nearly a century, seeing widespread use (particularly mixed with boric acid in Dakin's solution) during World War I. In subsequent decades, pediatric providers observed that patients with AD often improved in summer months, with exposure to sun and swimming pools.[60] Although providers have recommended bleach baths to patients with AD for decades, there was no high-quality evidence for their

efficacy until 2009, when a group of researchers at Northwestern University examined the effect of intranasal mupirocin plus dilute bleach baths on the EASI score in 31 pediatric patients with moderate to severe AD and evidence of infection.[61] In this study, patients were instructed to use one-half of a cup of 6% household bleach diluted in a full 40-gallon tub. Those assigned to the intervention group were instructed to bathe in the bleach bath twice a week for 5 to 10 minutes and apply intranasal mupirocin. Those in the control group were instructed to take plain water baths and use intranasal petrolatum. At 1 and 3 months, patients in the treatment group exhibited a significantly greater decrease in the EASI score than those in the control group, even though the proportion of patients with positive bacterial cultures at 3 months remained unchanged.[61] Subsequently, other researchers also investigated the effect of bleach baths on superinfection and AD severity. In particular, 3 other randomized, controlled trials have evaluated bleach baths between 2009 and 2018.[62–64] These subsequent studies used blinding, using unlabeled bottles of bleach or water, although the quality of blinding is questionable given that bleach has a distinct odor. One of these studies showed improved EASI scores and decreased percent body surface area with 2 months of bleach baths compared with water, but the other studies did not show any benefit to bleach baths. Hon and colleagues,[62] writing in 2016, found in a double-blind randomized, controlled trial that there was no benefit with bleach baths for most outcomes examined and a greater improvement in percent body surface area involvement with plain water baths. A 2018 metaanalysis of these studies found that, overall, there was no benefit to bleach baths over plain water baths, although large, well-designed studies examining the efficacy of bleach baths are lacking.[65] This metaanalysis also raised the potential issue of asthma exacerbations in some patients who take bleach baths. Although no report of asthma exacerbation owing to bleach bath has been published as of this writing, pool workers and swimmers are known from epidemiologic studies to have higher asthma incidence, suggesting that chlorine may be irritating to the bronchi in susceptible individuals.[66] One of the authors of the metaanalysis reported anecdotal experience with patients taking bleach baths who experienced asthma exacerbations from bleach bath fumes.[65]

This metaanalysis might indicate that hydration followed by emollient application is what underlies the improvement seen in those who benefit from bleach baths, rather than the effect of bleach itself. However, it may also indicate that studies were not sufficiently powered to demonstrate the benefit of bleach baths. For the time being, many practitioners continue to recommend bleach baths in their clinical practice because it is an inexpensive intervention that many patients report to be enjoyable and beneficial.

SYSTEMIC THERAPIES

In 2017, the International Eczema Council released expert recommendations on the appropriate use of systemic therapy. Systemic therapy can be highly effective for patients with AD, but traditional immune suppressant therapy (such as cyclosporine A) is associated with significant adverse events. The new biologic agent dupilumab has a favorable adverse event profile, with a wholesale acquisition cost of $37,000 per year. Given the risks and costs associated with systemic therapy, providers should carefully ascertain the diagnosis of AD before starting treatment. In the 2017 International Eczema Council guidelines, the panel acknowledged the number of conditions that may resemble AD and recommended careful consideration of alternate diagnoses before initiating systemic therapy. Such consideration could include careful history and examination alone, or biopsy, KOH prep, microscopy for scabies mites, and/or patch testing, depending on the clinical picture. Oral cyclosporine, methotrexate, and mycophenolate mofetil, along with other systemic immune suppressants, remain as treatment options for severe or refractory disease. However, these treatments carry significant adverse effects. Newer agents are actively being investigated in the treatment of severe AD.

Dupilumab

Dupilumab, a human monoclonal antibody to the IL-4α subunit in IL-4 and IL-13, has shown promising results in studies of asthma and AD. In a phase IIb randomized trial involving 379 adult patients with moderate to severe AD, a dose-dependent relationship was seen, with a 74% decrease in the EASI after 16 weeks of treatment with dupilumab 300 mg once a week and a 68% decrease in the EASI with treatment every 2 weeks at this dose.[67] Dupilumab has also been shown to improve patient-oriented outcomes, particularly health-related quality of life, pruritus, and sleep quality.[67] In the subsequent phase III SOLO1 and 2 trials, EASI-75, 37% to 38% of study subjects receiving weekly dupilumab achieved the primary endpoint of IGA clear or almost clear with at least a 2-point decrease from baseline at the end of 16 weeks of therapy, compared with 10% of patients in the placebo group.[68] The LIBERTY AD CHRONOS trial was designed to evaluate the long-term safety and efficacy of dupilumab.[69] Subjects received dupilumab 300 mg weekly or twice weekly, or placebo. Thirty-nine percent of patients in the dupilumab groups, compared with 12% of patients in the placebo group, achieved the primary endpoint of IGA clear/almost clear at week 52, with a 2-point or greater decrease compared with baseline. Patients in the dupilumab groups were found to be more likely to develop noninfectious conjunctivitis, whose etiology is the subject of continued investigation, speculation, and debate.[70]

THERAPEUTIC EDUCATION

Therapeutic patient education (TPE) refers to the transfer of skills and information related to a patient's disease. The purpose of TPE is to both provide the tools needed for patients to self-manage their disease between health care provider visits, as well as a sense of self-efficacy related to the patient's disease state. TPE has been successfully implemented in a number of chronic diseases, including congestive heart failure,[71] diabetes mellitus,[72,73] cancer,[74] rheumatoid arthritis,[75] human immunodeficiency virus infection,[76] chronic pain,[77] and stroke-induced neurologic deficits.[78] In these disease states, high-quality evidence in the form of randomized trials exists showing that TPE improves a number of disease-related outcomes as well as measures of overall well-being. By comparison, TPE in AD is a relatively less established and large, randomized trials are lacking. One simple way to implement TPE is through a personalized, written eczema action plan. One randomized trial tested the effect of written eczema action plan compared with standard verbal instruction in 37 patients. The use of a written eczema action plan resulted in improved subject understanding of treatment plan, medication risks and benefits, anatomic location of medication use, and duration of treatment.[79] Materials for TPE in AD have been developed, as well as recommendations for their implementation, primarily by European practitioners. Although TPE for AD is not yet widely implemented in North America, such materials provide a starting point for practitioners who are interested in TPE. TPE is a low-risk intervention that seems to be effective in many chronic disease states, and limited evidence in AD suggests it potentially may benefit families who have long struggled with this disease.

REFERENCES

1. Silverberg NB, Silverberg JI. Inside out or outside in: does atopic dermatitis disrupt barrier function or

does disruption of barrier function trigger atopic dermatitis? Cutis 2015;96(6):359–61.

2. Kim HJ, Baek J, Lee JR, et al. Optimization of cytokine milieu to reproduce atopic dermatitis-related gene expression in HaCaT keratinocyte cell line. Immune Netw 2018;18(1):e9.

3. Brunner PM, Leung DYM, Guttman-Yassky E. Immunologic, microbial, and epithelial interactions in atopic dermatitis. Ann Allergy Asthma Immunol 2018;120(1):34–41.

4. Honzke S, Wallmeyer L, Ostrowski A, et al. Influence of Th2 cytokines on the cornified envelope, tight junction proteins, and ss-defensins in filaggrin-deficient skin equivalents. J Invest Dermatol 2016; 136(3):631–9.

5. Kelleher M, Dunn-Galvin A, Hourihane JOB, et al. Skin barrier dysfunction measured by transepidermal water loss at 2 days and 2 months predates and predicts atopic dermatitis at 1 year. J Allergy Clin Immunol 2015;135(4):930–5.e1.

6. Horimukai K, Morita K, Narita M, et al. Transepidermal water loss measurement during infancy can predict the subsequent development of atopic dermatitis regardless of filaggrin mutations. Allergol Int 2016;65(1):103–8.

7. Berents TL, Carlsen KCL, Mowinckel P, et al. Transepidermal water loss in infancy associated with atopic eczema at 2 years of age: a population-based cohort study. Br J Dermatol 2017;177(3):e35–7.

8. Lee MY, Lee DSY, Lee SH, et al. Additive effect between prenatal depression and transepidermal water loss on atopic dermatitis via Th2 immune responses: COCOA study. J Allergy Clin Immunol 2018;141(2, Supplement):AB232.

9. Schultz Larsen F. Atopic dermatitis: a genetic-epidemiologic study in a population-based twin sample. J Am Acad Dermatol 1993;28(5 Pt 1): 719–23.

10. Thomsen SF, Elmose C, Szecsi PB, et al. Filaggrin gene loss-of-function mutations explain discordance of atopic dermatitis within dizygotic twin pairs. Int J Dermatol 2016;55(12):1341–4.

11. Irvine AD, McLean WH, Leung DY. Filaggrin mutations associated with skin and allergic diseases. N Engl J Med 2011;365(14):1315–27.

12. Margolis DJ, Gupta J, Apter AJ, et al. Filaggrin-2 variation is associated with more persistent atopic dermatitis in African American subjects. J Allergy Clin Immunol 2014;133(3):784–9.

13. Winge MC, Bilcha KD, Lieden A, et al. Novel filaggrin mutation but no other loss-of-function variants found in Ethiopian patients with atopic dermatitis. Br J Dermatol 2011;165(5):1074–80.

14. Margolis DJ, Apter AJ, Gupta J, et al. The persistence of atopic dermatitis and filaggrin (FLG) mutations in a US longitudinal cohort. J Allergy Clin Immunol 2012;130(4):912–7.

15. Ma CA, Stinson JR, Zhang Y, et al. Germline hypomorphic CARD11 mutations in severe atopic disease. Nat Genet 2017;49(8):1192–201.

16. Williams MR, Gallo RL. The role of the skin microbiome in atopic dermatitis. Curr Allergy Asthma Rep 2015;15(11):65.

17. Koliada A, Syzenko G, Moseiko V, et al. Association between body mass index and Firmicutes/Bacteroidetes ratio in an adult Ukrainian population. BMC Microbiol 2017;17:120.

18. Christianson A. 4 Ways to get firm and cute by lowering firmicutes. The Huffington Post; 2014.

19. Sugimoto S, Iwamoto T, Takada K, et al. Staphylococcus epidermidis Esp degrades specific proteins associated with Staphylococcus aureus biofilm formation and host-pathogen interaction. J Bacteriol 2013;195(8):1645–55.

20. Nakatsuji T, Chen TH, Narala S, et al. Antimicrobials from human skin commensal bacteria protect against Staphylococcus aureus and are deficient in atopic dermatitis. Sci Transl Med 2017;9(378) [pii:eaah4680].

21. Myles IA, Earland NJ, Anderson ED, et al. First-in-human topical microbiome transplantation with Roseomonas mucosa for atopic dermatitis. JCI Insight 2018;3(9) [pii: 120608].

22. Krämer U, Lemmen CH, Behrendt H, et al. The effect of environmental tobacco smoke on eczema and allergic sensitization in children. Br J Dermatol 2004;150(1):111–8.

23. Patrizi A, Raone B, Ravaioli GM. Management of atopic dermatitis: safety and efficacy of phototherapy. Clin Cosmet Investig Dermatol 2015;8:511–20.

24. Langan SM, Bourke JF, Silcocks P, et al. An exploratory prospective observational study of environmental factors exacerbating atopic eczema in children. Br J Dermatol 2006;154(5):979–80.

25. Paternoster L, Savenije OE, Heron J, et al. Identification of atopic dermatitis subgroups in children from 2 longitudinal birth cohorts. J Allergy Clin Immunol 2018;141(3):964–71.

26. Simpson EL, Bieber T, Eckert L, et al. Patient burden of moderate to severe atopic dermatitis (AD): insights from a phase 2b clinical trial of dupilumab in adults. J Am Acad Dermatol 2016;74(3):491–8.

27. Vakharia PP, Chopra R, Sacotte R, et al. Burden of skin pain in atopic dermatitis. Ann Allergy Asthma Immunol 2017;119(6):548–52.e3.

28. Holgate ST. The epithelium takes centre stage in asthma and atopic dermatitis. Trends Immunol 2007;28(6):248–51.

29. Jackson P, Baker R, Lessof M, et al. Intestinal permeability in patients with eczema and food allergy. Lancet 1981;317(8233):1285–6.

30. Groot AC. The frequency of contact allergy in atopic patients with dermatitis. Contact Dermatitis 1990; 22(5):273–7.

31. Zheng T, Yu J, Oh MH, et al. The atopic march: progression from atopic dermatitis to allergic rhinitis and asthma. Allergy Asthma Immunol Res 2011; 3(2):67–73.
32. Yaghmaie P, Koudelka CW, Simpson EL. Mental health comorbidity in patients with atopic dermatitis. J Allergy Clin Immunol 2013;131(2):428–33.
33. Buske-Kirschbaum A, Schmitt J, Plessow F, et al. Psychoendocrine and psychoneuroimmunological mechanisms in the comorbidity of atopic eczema and attention deficit/hyperactivity disorder. Psychoneuroendocrinology 2013;38(1):12–23.
34. Gómez RL, Edgin JO. Sleep as a window into early neural development: shifts in sleep-dependent learning effects across early childhood. Child Dev Perspect 2015;9(3):183–9.
35. Schmitt J, Buske-Kirschbaum A, Tesch F, et al. Increased attention-deficit/hyperactivity symptoms in atopic dermatitis are associated with history of antihistamine use. Allergy 2018;73(3):615–26.
36. Nicholas MN, Gooderham MJ. Atopic dermatitis, depression, and suicidality. J Cutan Med Surg 2017;21(3):237–42.
37. Holm JG, Agner T, Clausen ML, et al. Quality of life and disease severity in patients with atopic dermatitis. J Eur Acad Dermatol Venereol 2016;30(10):1760–7.
38. Dalgard FJ, Gieler U, Tomas-Aragones L, et al. The psychological burden of skin diseases: a cross-sectional multicenter study among dermatological out-patients in 13 European countries. J Invest Dermatol 2015;135(4):984–91.
39. Silverberg JI, Kleiman E, Lev-Tov H, et al. Association between obesity and atopic dermatitis in childhood: a case-control study. J Allergy Clin Immunol 2011;127(5):1180–6.e1.
40. Silverberg J, Silverberg N, Lee-Wong M. Association between atopic dermatitis and obesity in adulthood. Br J Dermatol 2012;166(3):498–504.
41. Olesen AB, Juul S, Birkebæk N, et al. Association between atopic dermatitis and insulin-dependent diabetes mellitus: a case-control study. Lancet 2001;357(9270):1749–52.
42. Simpson EL, Berry TM, Brown PA, et al. A pilot study of emollient therapy for the primary prevention of atopic dermatitis. J Am Acad Dermatol 2010;63(4):587–93.
43. Simpson EL, Chalmers JR, Hanifin JM, et al. Emollient enhancement of the skin barrier from birth offers effective atopic dermatitis prevention. J Allergy Clin Immunol 2014;134(4):818–23.
44. Sicherer SH, Sampson HA, Eichenfield LF, Rotrosen D. The Benefits of New Guidelines to Prevent Peanut Allergy. Pediatrics 2017;139(6). pii: e20164293.
45. Du Toit G, Roberts G, Sayre PH, et al. Randomized trial of peanut consumption in infants at risk for peanut allergy. N Engl J Med 2015;372(9):803–13.
46. Du Toit G, Sayre PH, Roberts G, et al. Effect of avoidance on peanut allergy after early peanut consumption. N Engl J Med 2016;374(15):1435–43.
47. Togias A, Cooper SF, Acebal ML, et al. Addendum guidelines for the prevention of peanut allergy in the United States: report of the National Institute of Allergy and Infectious Diseases-sponsored expert panel. Allergy Asthma Clin Immunol 2017;13(1):1.
48. Salter H. On some points in the treatment and clinical history of asthma. Edinb Med J 1859;4(12):1109.
49. Choi OH, Shamim MT, Padgett WL, et al. Caffeine and theophylline analogues: correlation of behavioral effects with activity as adenosine receptor antagonists and as phosphodiesterase inhibitors. Life Sci 1988;43(5):387–98.
50. Wittmann M, Helliwell PS. Phosphodiesterase 4 inhibition in the treatment of psoriasis, psoriatic arthritis and other chronic inflammatory diseases. Dermatol Ther 2013;3(1):1–15.
51. Paller AS, Tom WL, Lebwohl MG, et al. Efficacy and safety of crisaborole ointment, a novel, nonsteroidal phosphodiesterase 4 (PDE4) inhibitor for the topical treatment of atopic dermatitis (AD) in children and adults. J Am Acad Dermatol 2016;75(3):494–503.e6.
52. Eichenfield LF, Call RS, Forsha DW, et al. Long-term safety of crisaborole ointment 2% in children and adults with mild to moderate atopic dermatitis. J Am Acad Dermatol 2017;77(4):641–9.e5.
53. Hanifin JM, Ellis CN, Frieden IJ, et al. OPA-15406, a novel, topical, nonsteroidal, selective phosphodiesterase-4 (PDE4) inhibitor, in the treatment of adult and adolescent patients with mild to moderate atopic dermatitis (AD): a phase-II randomized, double-blind, placebo-controlled study. J Am Acad Dermatol 2016;75(2):297–305.
54. Ohba F, Matsuki S, Imayama S, et al. Efficacy of a novel phosphodiesterase inhibitor, E6005, in patients with atopic dermatitis: an investigator-blinded, vehicle-controlled study. J Dermatolog Treat 2016;27(5):467–72.
55. Bao L, Zhang H, Chan LS. The involvement of the JAK-STAT signaling pathway in chronic inflammatory skin disease atopic dermatitis. JAKSTAT 2013;2(3):e24137.
56. Bissonnette R, Papp KA, Poulin Y, et al. Topical tofacitinib for atopic dermatitis: a phase IIa randomized trial. Br J Dermatol 2016;175(5):902–11.
57. Cotter DG, Schairer D, Eichenfield L. Emerging therapies for atopic dermatitis: JAK inhibitors. J Am Acad Dermatol 2018;78(3S1):S53–62.
58. Nakagawa H, Nemoto O, Igarashi A, et al. Efficacy and safety of topical JTE-052, a Janus kinase inhibitor, in Japanese adult patients with moderate-to-severe atopic dermatitis: a phase II, multicentre, randomized, vehicle-controlled clinical study. Br J Dermatol 2018;178(2):424–32.

59. Peppers J, Paller AS, Maeda-Chubachi T, et al. A phase 2, randomized dose-finding study of tapinarof (GSK2894512 Cream) for the treatment of atopic dermatitis. J Am Acad Dermatol 2018.

60. History: history of bleach baths. BleachBath.org - A safe solution for compromised skin 2016. Available at: http://www.bleachbath.com/how-it-works/history/. Accessed May 1, 2018.

61. Huang JT, Abrams M, Tlougan B, et al. Treatment of Staphylococcus aureus colonization in atopic dermatitis decreases disease severity. Pediatrics 2009;123(5):e808–14.

62. Hon K, Tsang Y, Lee V, et al. Efficacy of sodium hypochlorite (bleach) baths to reduce Staphylococcus aureus colonization in childhood onset moderate-to-severe eczema: a randomized, placebo-controlled cross-over trial. J Dermatolog Treat 2016;27(2): 156–62.

63. Gonzalez ME, Schaffer JV, Orlow SJ, et al. Cutaneous microbiome effects of fluticasone propionate cream and adjunctive bleach baths in childhood atopic dermatitis. J Am Acad Dermatol 2016;75(3): 481–93.e8.

64. Wong SM, Ng TG, Baba R. Efficacy and safety of sodium hypochlorite (bleach) baths in patients with moderate to severe atopic dermatitis in Malaysia. J Dermatol 2013;40(11):874–80.

65. Chopra R, Vakharia PP, Sacotte R, et al. Efficacy of bleach baths in reducing severity of atopic dermatitis: a systematic review and meta-analysis. Ann Allergy asthma Immunol 2017;119(5):435–40.

66. Thickett K, McCoach J, Gerber J, et al. Occupational asthma caused by chloramines in indoor swimming-pool air. Eur Respir J 2002;19(5):827–32.

67. Simpson EL, Gadkari A, Worm M, et al. Dupilumab therapy provides clinically meaningful improvement in patient-reported outcomes (PROs): a phase IIb, randomized, placebo-controlled, clinical trial in adult patients with moderate to severe atopic dermatitis (AD). J Am Acad Dermatol 2016;75(3):506–15.

68. Simpson EL, Bieber T, Guttman-Yassky E, et al. Two phase 3 trials of dupilumab versus placebo in atopic dermatitis. N Engl J Med 2016;375(24):2335–48.

69. Blauvelt A, de Bruin-Weller M, Gooderham M, et al. Long-term management of moderate-to-severe atopic dermatitis with dupilumab and concomitant topical corticosteroids (LIBERTY AD CHRONOS): a 1-year, randomised, double-blinded, placebo-controlled, phase 3 trial. Lancet 2017;389(10086): 2287–303.

70. de Bruin-Weller M, Graham NMH, Pirozzi G, et al. Could conjunctivitis in patients with atopic dermatitis treated with dupilumab be caused by colonization with Demodex and increased interleukin-17 levels? Reply from the authors. Br J Dermatol 2018;178(5): 1220–1.

71. Albano MG, Jourdain P, De Andrade V, et al. Therapeutic patient education in heart failure: do studies provide sufficient information about the educational programme? Arch Cardiovasc Dis 2014;107(5): 328–39.

72. Golay A, Lagger G, Chambouleyron M, et al. Therapeutic education of diabetic patients. Diabetes Metab Res Rev 2008;24(3):192–6.

73. Jansa M, Vidal M, Conget I, et al. Therapeutic education regarding type 1 diabetes (DM1). Rev Enferm 2007;30(10):23–32 [in Spanish].

74. Arthurs G, Simpson J, Brown A, et al. The effectiveness of therapeutic patient education on adherence to oral anti-cancer medicines in adult cancer patients in ambulatory care settings: a systematic review. JBI Database System Rev Implement Rep 2015;13(5):244–92.

75. Perdriger A, Michinov E. Therapeutic patient education: from infantilization to critical thinking. Joint Bone Spine 2015;82(5):299–301.

76. Njom Nlend AE, Lyeb AS, Moyo S, et al. Therapeutic patient education and disclosure of status of HIV infected children in Yaounde, Cameroon Achievements and competence. Med Sante Trop 2016; 26(3):308–11.

77. Gross A, Forget M, St George K, et al. Patient education for neck pain. Cochrane Database Syst Rev 2012;(3):CD005106.

78. Daviet JC, Bonan I, Caire JM, et al. Therapeutic patient education for stroke survivors: non-pharmacological management. A literature review. Ann Phys Rehabil Med 2012;55(9–10):641–56.

79. Shi VY, Nanda S, Lee K, et al. Improving patient education with an eczema action plan: a randomized controlled trial. JAMA Dermatol 2013;149(4):481–3.

Contact Dermatitis
Emerging Trends

Emily C. Milam, MD*, David E. Cohen, MD, MPH

KEYWORDS

- Allergic contact dermatitis • Irritant contact dermatitis • Contact allergen • Patch testing
- Surfactants • Preservatives • Acrylates • Fragrances

KEY POINTS

- Contact dermatitis is a commonly encountered diagnosis in dermatology.
- Trends in allergic contact dermatitis are influenced by industrial practices and consumer behaviors.
- Successful diagnosis of contact dermatitis relies on awareness of existing trends and relevant allergens.
- There are many emerging contact allergens, including surfactants such as alkyl glucosides, the fragrances linalool and D-limonene, the preservative methylisothiazolinone, the metal cobalt, and propylene glycol.

INTRODUCTION

Contact dermatitis is a commonly encountered diagnosis in dermatology. Exposure to the natural and synthetic chemicals of everyday life, whether from consumer products, occupational settings, or personal diversions, can trigger a variety of irritant or allergic eruptions in susceptible hosts. Cutaneous manifestations of contact dermatitis depend on the chemical, the duration and nature of contact, and the susceptibility of the exposed individual. Awareness of emerging chemicals is essential to the successful diagnosis of allergic and irritant contact dermatoses, which are prevalent conditions that confer significant emotional, social, economic, and occupational burdens.

Trends in allergen exposure are constantly evolving and can vary by region. Although some allergens' clinical importance escalates over time, others become less relevant due to decreased usage. Certain allergens continue to dominate the list of most common offenders: nickel remains the most common allergen positive on patch testing worldwide. Industrial settings and consumer goods frequently introduce new chemicals, such as methylisothiazolinone, resulting in shifts in allergen exposure and sensitization. Diligent observation of these trends allows dermatologists to identify new, relevant contact irritants and allergens.

The realm of contact dermatitis is complex. This article aims to distill the most recent and noteworthy trends within the field, organized by allergen category, with particular attention to newer and/or controversial allergens.

SURFACTANTS

Surfactants reduce the surface tension of proteins and lipids of the stratum corneum, aiding in removal of skin debris such as sebum, oil, and dirt. These properties of surfactants are used in a variety of leave-on and rinse-off cosmetics, including shower gels, shampoos, moisturizers, sunscreens, deodorants, mousses, fragrances, and baby wipes, among many other products.

Disclosures: The authors do not have any relevant disclosures or conflicts of interest.
The Ronald O. Perelman Department of Dermatology, New York University School of Medicine, 240 East 38th Street, Floor 11, New York, NY 10016, USA
* Corresponding author.
E-mail address: Emily.Milam@nyulangone.org

Dermatol Clin 37 (2019) 21–28
https://doi.org/10.1016/j.det.2018.07.005

Although rinse-off products have transient contact with the skin, certain components can bind strongly to the stratum corneum and trigger irritation or allergy.

Increased attention to surfactants' sensitizing potential was noted in 2004, when cocamidopropyl betaine (CAPB) was declared the American Contact Dermatitis Society (ACDS) allergen of the year (Table 1).[1] CAPB, well known for its use in many baby and gentle shampoos, is incorporated into many consumer products including body washes, toothpastes, makeup removers, and contact lens solutions. Cases of contact allergy from CAPB emerged as early as 1983; however, later studies suggested that the contaminants of CAPB, namely dimethylaminopropylamine and amidoamine, were largely to blame.[2]

More recently, alkyl glucosides, a botanic and biodegradable family of relatively gentle surfactants, have been "rediscovered," becoming increasingly popular in ecofriendly consumer products.[3,4] With this, increased rates of sensitization to surfactants have been observed. Alkyl glucoside became allergen of the year in 2017.[5]

Although alkyl glucoside has been available for more than 40 years, its use has burgeoned over the last 2 decades. Alkyl surfactants are derived from the condensation of renewable, biodegradable, and plant-based ingredients such as palm, coconut, and rapeseed oil (which provide fatty alcohols) and corn, wheat starch, and potato (which provide glucose). They have been incorporated into numerous consumer products, which tout its natural appeal. Beyond their environmental allure, alkyl glucosides are also milder, more stable, and require lower concentrations for efficacy compared with other surfactants.

Although alkyl glucosides are generally considered to be of low irritancy and allergenicity, particularly when compared with the more irritating anionic surfactants sodium lauryl sulfate and sodium laureth sulfate, their increased use has sparked an increase in sensitization. Goossens and colleagues[6] reported the first 2 cases of contact allergy to alkyl glucosides found in cosmetic and cleansing products in 2003.

Decyl glucoside is a "hidden" allergen in the sunscreen ingredient Tinosorb M (which is not yet approved for use in the United States by the Food and Drug Administration [FDA]). In 2011, the Voluntary Cosmetic Registration Program database reported that decyl glucoside was an ingredient in 492 cosmetics, mainly rinse-off products.[7] As a result of increased reports of sensitivity to decyl glucoside, it was introduced to the North American Contact Dermatitis Group (NACDG) standard patch testing series in 2009, at a 5% concentration in petrolatum. The rate of positive patch test reactions to decyl glucoside has increased from 1.3% in 2014 to 2.2% in 2016.[4] Patch testing for such surfactants can prove challenging, because they are tested at irritant concentrations. Strong positive reactions are thought to reflect actual sensitization.

ACRYLATES

Acrylates are a class of glues, adhesives, synthetic plastics, and resins that are used in innumerable products owing to their durable and inert properties. Plexiglass, a transparent safety glass made of polymethyl methacrylate, is a well-known example of an acrylate. Acrylates are found in medical devices (dental implants/prosthesis, contact lenses, bone cement, wound dressings, and surgical glues), aesthetics (eyelash and hair extensions, nail lacquers), and industrial products (plastics, glues, adhesives, paints, printing inks, and fiberglass).[8]

Acrylates are derived from acrylic or methacrylic acid monomers, which are potently volatile irritants and sensitizers. Once the unstable acrylate monomers polymerize (either spontaneously or on ultraviolet light exposure), they become more innocuous. Although acrylate hypersensitivity is relatively uncommon, it is an important cause of

Table 1	
American Contact Dermatitis Society allergens of the year	
2018	Propylene glycol
2017	Alkyl glucosides
2016	Cobalt
2015	Formaldehyde
2014	Benzophenones
2013	Methylisothiazolinone
2012	Acrylate
2011	Dimethyl fumarate
2010	Neomycin
2009	Mixed dialkyl thiourea
2008	Nickel
2007	Fragrance
2006	p-Phenylenediamine
2005	Corticosteroids
2004	Cocamidopropyl betaine
2003	Bacitracin
2002	Thimerosal
2001	Gold
2000	Disperse blue dyes

Data from Refs.[3,58,70]

contact dermatitis. The earliest case reports of contact dermatitis to acrylates first appeared in the 1940s, when Stevenson and Moody each reported a case of occupational contact dermatitis in a dental technician.[9,10]

Historically, contact dermatitis from acrylates, particularly methyl methacrylate, was focused within occupational settings, including dentistry, orthopedic surgery, aeronautics, and printing industries.[11] However, the incorporation of acrylates in cosmetic products, particularly artificial nails, "shellac," lacquers, and related items, has lead to a shift in acrylate sensitization to beauticians and artificial nail consumers.[12,13] A recent 2018 study by Gonçalo and colleagues[14] demonstrated that 67.3% cases of positive patch test reactions to acrylates were attributable to nail aesthetics. Another group reported nails to be the culprit in 85.2% of positive tests among 54 patients.[15]

Nail technicians and consumers are at especially high risk for acrylate sensitization because they are directly exposed to (meth)acrylate in their unstable monomer form (before being stabilized by ultraviolet light exposure). Nail-related allergic contact dermatitis (ACD) from acrylates typically manifests as hand eczema, often with periungual involvement. Onycholysis, onychodystrophy, and fingertip paraesthesias can also be seen.[13] Ectopic areas of involvement on the face and arms may result from airborne exposure to dust generated by nail sculpting, evaporation of acrylate monomers, or by transfer from contaminated surfaces or hands.[11]

Patch testing for acrylates can be difficult, as the acrylate preparations are volatile and may evaporate from the chamber during storage, reducing patch test concentrations at the time of testing, which can lead to false-negative results.[8,16,17] When patch tested, acrylate-allergic patients often display multiple positive tests, representing either cross-reactions or the presence of impurities not disclosed in material safety data sheets. The NACDG standard series includes methyl methacrylate, ethyl acrylate, and 2-hydroxyethyl methacrylate, which collectively seem to be sufficient for screening allergens in most cases.[17] However, clinicians should remain vigilant for acrylate allergy even if initial screening is negative and consider an expanded panel of test chemicals, including ethyl acrylate, ethylene dimethacrylate, triethylene glycol diacrylate, and ethyl cyanoacrylate. Protective measures such as using gloves can be helpful; however, (meth)acrylates can permeate glove material even after brief exposure. Nitrile gloves confer better protection than latex.[18] Of note, absorbent dressings and wound care products have also been implicated as a newly emerging source of (meth)acrylate contact dermatitis.[19]

FRAGRANCES

Fragrances, a group of naturally derived and synthetic chemicals defined by their odor-enhancing or odor-blending properties, are incorporated into numerous food, industrial, clothing, cosmetic, and hygienic products.[20,21] Although relatively innocuous chemicals overall, fragrances are the second most common cause of positive patch test results in the general population, after nickel.[22] Within consumers of cosmetic products, fragrances represent the most common cause of ACD,[23] affecting 1% to 8% of the adult population, particularly middle-aged women.[24–26]

A recent United Kingdom study from 1996 to 2015 found a 47-time higher incidence rate ratio of allergy to fragrance in beauticians, hairdressers, and those working in related occupations compared with all other reference occupations combined.[27] Perfumes can have upward of 100 different chemicals, many of which have sensitizing potential.[28] Notably, new fragrance allergens can be hidden ingredients on cosmetic and cleansing products, even those that describe themselves as "fragrance free."

Fragrance mix I (FMI) was developed in 1977 by Larsen and was the most important screening marker for contact allergy to fragrances for decades.[28] FMI consists of 8 fragrance chemicals (amyl cinnamal, cinnamyl alcohol, cinnamal, eugenol, geraniol, hydroxycitronellal isoeugenol, and *Evernia prunastri* [oakmoss absolute]). Although these 8 chemicals continue to be relevant fragrance allergens to this day, a need for an expanded panel was recognized in the 1990s, when research suggested that 15% of relevant perfume allergies were not identified by FMI.[29] In 2005, fragrance mixed II was introduced—including the chemicals Lyral, citral, citronellol, farnesol, coumarin, and hexyl-cinnamic aldehyde—which effectively identified additional patients with fragrance sensitivities missed by FMI.[30] However, as perfumery practices and exposure patterns continue to evolve, there is a new emerging cohort of fragrance-allergenic patients who are not being successfully identified by either fragrance mix panels.

Two emergent fragrance allergens are linalool and limonene, which are terpenes with a fresh, flowery or citrus odor and solvent properties. Although weakly allergenic in their pure forms, they can autooxidize into more potent hydroperoxide byproducts.[31] On exposure to air, both linalool and limonene readily oxidize into their more allergenic forms. This is relevant given their use in commercially available fragrances, which are delivered to the skin by aerosolization.[32] Linalool can be detected in 88% of essential oils, including lavender, ylang-ylang, and rosemary oils.[33] D-Limonene can be found in upward of 97% of essential oils, including tea tree oil.

Unfortunately, available screening panels such as FMI, fragrance mix II, *Myroxylon pereirae* (balsam of Peru), and colophony fail to detect more than half of patients with linalool and D-limonene sensitivities.[34,35] Recently, the ACDS added lavender absolute, which contains linalool, to its Core Allergen Series; however, lavender is not a perfect proxy because the linalool is not delivered in its oxidized (and more allergenic) form.[36] *Nonoxidized* linalool and D-limonene rarely demonstrate positive patch tests reactions.[31,37] International studies have demonstrated that positive patch test findings for *oxidized* linalool and D-limonene, conversely, exceeds any other isolated fragrance allergens,[34,35,38] leading experts to call for their inclusion as separate allergens on patch testing.[31,39] This has fueled a growing consensus that the current screening fragrances are no longer sufficient to diagnose up-and-coming fragrance allergens.[38]

PRESERVATIVES

Preservatives are biocidal chemicals that inhibit growth of microorganisms and prevent putrefaction of foods, cosmetics, and industrial products. Preservatives have been responsible for several "contact allergy epidemics," dating back to the widespread use of formaldehyde in textiles and cosmetic products in the 1950s, methylchloroisothiazolinone/methylisothiazolinone (MCI/MI; trade names: Kathon G, Euxyl K 400) in the 1980s and, more recently, methyldibromo glutaronitrile (MDBGN) in the 1990s. Each of these epidemics has spawned policy change, and even the banning of MDBGN in European cosmetic products.[40]

Formaldehyde (or methanal) is a colorless, odorous gas created by incomplete combustion of wood, tobacco, coal, and gasoline. Formaldehyde has been incorporated into a wide range of products, including nail polish, personal hygiene products, wrinkle-free clothing, and Brazilian blowout treatments.

The use of formaldehyde has decreased over time owing to negative publicity of its carcinogenic and sensitizing effects. Formaldehyde-releasing preservatives (FRPs) were subsequently developed, with the idea that the amount of formaldehyde released would not be sufficient enough to cause a skin reaction. FRPs have essentially replaced formaldehyde in personal care products,

makeup, medications, and household cleaning products. According to the 2010 FDA Voluntary Cosmetic Registration Program database, FRPs could be found in approximately 20% of personal hygiene products and cosmetics (imidazolidinyl urea being the most common).[41] FRPs are present in 24% of leave-on products registered with the FDA, including 20% of moisturizers commercially available in the United States. The most relevant formaldehyde-releasing preservatives (listed in order of most to least releasing) are quaternium 15, diazolidinyl urea, dimethyl-dimethyl hydantoin, imidazolidinyl urea, and 2-bromo-2-nitropropane-1,3-diol (bronopol).

The preservative pair MCI/MI was later introduced in 1980 in a 3:1 combination. MCI/MI offered lower rates of sensitization than formaldehyde or FRPs, with less concern for toxicity. Soon after their introduction, rates of contact allergy to MCI/MI increased as high as 8% in some populations, catalyzing a new contact allergy epidemic.[42] Because MI was considered a weaker sensitizer than MCI, use of MI alone was approved for industrial and cosmetic products in 2000 and 2005, respectively.[43] With this, MI was increasingly incorporated into industrial and personal care products, with the number of MI-containing cosmetic products doubling between 2007 and 2010.[43] For example, MI was incorporated into moist toilet papers, instigating a wave of perianal dermatitis, and later into MI-containing makeup remover wipes, yielding many cases of eyelid dermatitis. The preservative methylisothiazolinone (MI) was thus named the ACDS contact allergen of the year in 2013.[43] MI alone is a less effective biocidal agent without MCI and therefore requires a higher (and more allergenic) concentration for effective use. Notably, a positive reaction to MI can be missed if a patient is patch tested only to the MCI/MI combination. The addition of MI alone, particularly at a concentration of 2000 ppm, greatly increases detection of MI sensitization.[44]

Parabens, the family of preservatives derived from the esters of parahydroxybenzoic acid, are incorporated into foods and cosmetics for their antimicrobial effects. Like many of the aforementioned preservatives, they are favored ingredients because they are inexpensive, odorless, and colorless. Parabens are far less sensitizing than other preservatives; the NACDG reports rates of ACD between 0.6% and 1.4%.[45] Moreover, ACD to parabens seems to occur most frequently on application to areas of skin breakdown. In fact, patients sensitized to parabens are often able to tolerate paraben-containing products when applied to normal skin, a phenomenon that has been coined the "paraben paradox."[46]

Despite proving themselves as weak allergens with decades of supportive patch testing data, concerns related to parabens have escalated due to increased media coverage that called their safety into question. Because parabens demonstrate weak estrogenic activity in vitro and in animal models, a suggestion of their role as "endocrine disruptors" exploded in popular press, raising alarm that parabens cause breast cancer or reproductive abnormalities. However, follow-up studies have failed to validate their role in hormonal aberrations or infertility. Nonetheless, "paraben-free" is now emblazoned across many consumer products. Unfortunately, the preservatives tasked with replacing parabens, such as methylisothiazolinone, are actually more allergenic than parabens and are likely driving the recent increase in ACD, as just discussed.[47,48]

METALS

Metals represent a common class of contact allergens in both occupational and nonoccupational settings. Gold was the first metal to be designated contact allergen of the year in 2001,[49] however, not without controversy. The clinical relevance of positive patch tests to gold sodium thiosulfate (as it is tested) and the interpretation of these results are disputed. Many patients with positive patch tests to gold do not necessarily react to direct contact with gold jewelry. Some have pointed to impurities in gold jewelry, such as cobalt, as being the true culprits. As such, ACDS has stated that patients with a positive patch test to gold but without dermatitis on environmental gold exposure can be considered to have an irrelevant sensitization.[50]

Nickel was the next metal to be designated as allergen of the year in 2008. Nickel can be found in innumerable items including jewelry, clothing buckles and buttons, electronics (such as cell phones and tablets), doorknobs, multivitamins, food—the list continues. Rates of nickel sensitization remain unparalleled. Patch testing data collected by the NACDG between 1992 and 2004 show a steady increase in nickel sensitivity, from 14.5% in 1992 to 18.8% in 2004 ($P<.0001$).[51] Among US children, rates of sensitization reached 28.1%, according to NACDG patch testing data from 2005 to 2012.[52] Body piercings are a likely source of exposure. The number of positive tests to nickel seems to increase linearly with the number of piercings (14.3% for 1 piercing to 34.0% with ≥5 piercings).[53]

In recent years, cobalt has surfaced as another metal with high sensitizing potential, earning the status of contact allergen of the year in 2016.[54]

Cobalt is often alloyed with other metals to enhance hardness and strength and can be found in jewelry, vehicle engines, magnets, cosmetics, clothing snaps and buttons, construction materials, orthopedic implants, medical devices, ceramics, cements, and even in some plastics and leather products. Rates of contact sensitization to cobalt are estimated to be 5.23%, with female gender doubling the risk of sensitization.[55] Prior dogmas suggested that cobalt allergy co-occurs with nickel or chromate allergy; however recent data disprove this dogma. Unpublished data (Fowler, 2016) from the NACDG indicate that 40% of patients positive to cobalt were actually negative to nickel.[54] Of note, a unique feature seen in cobalt patch-testing is the false-positive "poral" reaction, in which inflammation specifically arises within the skin's acrosyringium, giving a speckled irritant reaction.

PROPYLENE GLYCOL

Propylene glycol (PG) is a synthetic alcohol with emollient, solvent, antimicrobial, and emulsifying properties. PG is viscous, colorless, and has low toxicity with little smell or taste, making it a favorite ingredient in many cosmetics, personal hygiene products, medications (including topical corticosteroids), food products, and, more recently, electronic cigarettes.[56] Use of PG has expanded since its initial commercialization in the 1930s, and it is now present in more than 37% of the 4674 products logged in the ACDS's 2016 CAMP database.[57] PG was anointed the contact allergen of the year in 2018.[58]

Patch testing data suggest that PG sensitization rates range from 0.8% to 3.5%, depending on the testing concentration used (ie, 10% vs 30% in aqueous solution).[56,59,60] Contact dermatitis to PG is most often observed on the face, and systemic reactions can also be seen. Patch testing for PG and its relevance as a contact allergen is controversial. PG is a relatively weak sensitizer but an important irritant. As a result, the optimal patch-test concentration and timing of final readings are debated, because it can be difficult to distinguish true allergic reactions from irritant reactions. Moreover, weak hypersensitivity reactions can be mistakenly interpreted as insignificant.

The NACDG initially tested PG at 10% in aqueous solution; however in 1996 it increased the potency to 30% in aqueous solution. Later, in 2013, the NACDG added 100% PG to their standard screening tray.[61] Interpretation of results is multifaceted: reactions that are fast (<24 hours), with well-demarcated margins, or "decrescendo" in nature (presenting weekly at 48 hours, then dissipating by 96 hours) are all thought to be irritant reactions. Crescendo reactions, in which a stronger reaction is seen days later, around 96 hours, is thought to be more suggestive of true contact allergy.[62] Some experts suggest that any reaction to the 30% patch test concentration, whether allergic or irritant, has clinical relevance[57]; however, most of the products with such high concentrations of PG are washed-off and have very limited contact with the skin.

PARA-PHENYLENEDIAMINE

Para-phenylenediamine (PPD), the 2006 contact allergen of the year, is an aromatic amine that is a highly potent sensitizer and common cause of ACD. Typically sensitized individuals include hairdressers and consumers of hair dye, and henna tattoos, which can sensitize younger patients, compared with hair dye.[63] Hypersensitivity to PPD can manifest with an array of symptoms, ranging from pruritus, eczematous eruptions, and blisters to facial edema and even systemic reactions such as upper airway obstruction and myocarditis.[64] Prevalence of PPD sensitization is high, ranging from 1% to 6% of all patients with unspecified dermatitis, increasing from 38% to 97% in patients with suspected hair dye dermatitis.[65] Fortunately, new PPD-free hair dyes have emerged in the market and will hopefully reduce rates of ACD in this population.

DISCUSSION

The field of contact dermatitis is constantly evolving and expanding. Trends in ACD are shaped by the introduction of new chemicals, revival of older allergens, industrial practices, and consumer behaviors. A recent review by de Groot found that, on average, 17 newly described contact allergens causing ACD have been reported per year between 2008 and 2015, one-third of which are found in cosmetics.[66]

A common theme in modern-day contact dermatitis is the growing use of "ecofriendly" allergens, likely owing to consumers' increasing focus on nature-derived products. This popularity of hypoallergenic and natural products is shifting some of the burden of contact dermatitis from occupational workers to consumers. Similarly, new consumer fears of historically less allergenic ingredients, such as parabens, have catalyzed a shift toward use of "safer" chemicals, which are arguably no less toxic and in fact more potent sensitizers.

There is also increased attention on the co-occurrence of ACD among patients with atopic dermatitis (AD). Some available research suggests that children with compromised skin barriers should practice preemptive avoidance of potent allergens to mitigate risk of developing ACD. Perhaps supporting this theory, many of the aforementioned contact allergens—including CAPB, D-limonene, fragrances, surfactants, cobalt, and more—demonstrate relatively higher rates of sensitization among patients with AD compared with the general population.[55,67,68]

Another hot topic in contact dermatitis is how to assess for metal hypersensitivity in patients with implantable devices. Implantable devices include prosthetic joints, pacemakers, intrauterine devices, cardiovascular stents, and dental implants, among others. There are conflicting data and opinion on whether patients with known ACD to metals will tolerate implants and whether patients with implants and unexplained dermatitis warrant patch testing or, in extreme cases, device removal. The ACDS published its perspective in 2016, recommending presurgical patch testing only for patients with a clear self-reported metal sensitivity of severity significant enough to cause concern in the patient or health care provider. Although metal from an implanted device may cause sensitization, a positive patch test result does not prove symptom causality. When the history is uncertain and/or patch testing unavailable, the ACDS suggests use of titanium or oxinium-containing devices are preferable.[69]

As history demonstrates, new innovations and ever-changing consumer practices influence the emergence (or reemergence) of sensitizing chemicals. Successful diagnosis and management of contact dermatitis relies on awareness of these existing trends and relevant allergens.

REFERENCES

1. Fowler JF. Cocamidopropyl betaine. Dermatitis 2004;15(1):3–4.
2. Angelini G, Foti C, Rigano L, et al. 3-Dimethylaminopropylamine: a key substance in contact allergy to cocamidopropylbetaine? Contact Derm 1995;32(2):96–9.
3. Alfalah M, Loranger C, Sasseville D. Alkyl glucosides. Dermatitis 2017;28(1):3–4.
4. Loranger C, Alfalah M, Ferrier le bouedec MC, et al. Alkyl glucosides in contact dermatitis. Dermatitis 2017;28(1):5–13.
5. Sasseville D. Alkyl glucosides: 2017 "allergen of the year". Dermatitis 2017;28(4):296.
6. Goossens A, Decraene T, Platteaux N, et al. Glucosides as unexpected allergens in cosmetics. Contact Dermatitis 2003;48(3):164–6.

7. Fiume MM, Heldreth B, Bergfeld WF, et al. Safety assessment of decyl glucoside and other alkyl glucosides as used in cosmetics. Int J Toxicol 2013; 32(5 Suppl):22S–48S.

8. Sasseville D. Acrylates in contact dermatitis. Dermatitis 2012;23(1):6–16.

9. Stevenson WJ. Methyl methacrylate dermatitis. Contact Point 1941;18:171.

10. Moody WL. Severe reaction from acrylic liquid. Dent Dig 1941;47:305–7.

11. Geukens S, Goossens A. Occupational contact allergy to (meth)acrylates. Contact Derm 2001;44(3): 153–9.

12. Ramos L, Cabral R, Gonçalo M. Allergic contact dermatitis caused by acrylates and methacrylates– a 7-year study. Contact Derm 2014;71(2):102–7.

13. Raposo I, Lobo I, Amaro C, et al. Allergic contact dermatitis caused by (meth)acrylates in nail cosmetic products in users and nail technicians - a 5-year study. Contact Derm 2017;77(6):356–9.

14. Gonçalo M, Pinho A, Agner T, et al. Allergic contact dermatitis caused by nail acrylates in Europe. An EECDRG study. Contact Derm 2018;78(4):254–60.

15. Montgomery R, Stocks SJ, Wilkinson SM. Contact allergy resulting from the use of acrylate nails is increasing in both users and those who are occupationally exposed. Contact Derm 2016;74(2):120–2.

16. Mose KF, Andersen KE, Christensen LP. Stability of selected volatile contact allergens in different patch test chambers under different storage conditions. Contact Dermatitis 2012;66(4):172–9.

17. Drucker AM, Pratt MD. Acrylate contact allergy: patient characteristics and evaluation of screening allergens. Dermatitis 2011;22(2):98–101.

18. Andersson T, Bruze M, Björkner B. In vivo testing of the protection of gloves against acrylates in dentin-bonding systems on patients with known contact allergy to acrylates. Contact Derm 1999;41(5):254–9.

19. Spencer A, Gazzani P, Thompson DA. Acrylate and methacrylate contact allergy and allergic contact disease: a 13-year review. Contact Derm 2016; 75(3):157–64.

20. IFRA. Appendix 7 to the IFRA code of practice: definitions. 2006. Available at: http://www.ifraorg. org/. Accessed July 17, 2018.

21. Katsarou A, Armenaka M, Kalogeromitros D, et al. Contact reactions to fragrances. Ann Allergy Asthma Immunol 1999;82(5):449–55.

22. Cheng J, Zug KA. Fragrance allergic contact dermatitis. Dermatitis 2014;25(5):232–45.

23. Militello G, James W. Lyral: a fragrance allergen. Dermatitis 2005;16(1):41–4.

24. de Groot AC, Frosch PJ. Adverse reactions to fragrances. A clinical review. Contact Derm 1997; 36(2):57–86.

25. Van Oosten EJ, Schuttelaar MLA, Coenraads PJ. Clinical relevance of positive patch test reactions to the 26 EU-labelled fragrances. Contact Dermatitis 2009;61(4):217–23.

26. Johansen JD. Fragrance contact allergy—a clinical review. Am J Clin Dermatol 2003;4(11):789–98.

27. Montgomery RL, Agius R, Wilkinson SM, et al. UK trends of allergic occupational skin disease attributed to fragrances 1996-2015. Contact Derm 2018; 78(1):33–40.

28. Larsen WG. Perfume dermatitis. a study of 20 patients. Arch Dermatol 1977;113(5):623–6.

29. de Groot AC, van der Kley AMJ, Bruynzeel DP, et al. Frequency of false-negative reactions to the fragrance mix. Contact Dermatitis 1993;28:139–40.

30. Frosch PJ, Pirker C, Rastogi SC, et al. Patch testing with a new fragrance mix detects additional patients sensitive to perfumes and missed by the current fragrance mix. Contact Derm 2005;52(4): 207–15.

31. Nath NS, Liu B, Green C, et al. Contact allergy to hydroperoxides of linalool and D-limonene in a US population. Dermatitis 2017;28(5):313–6.

32. Sköld M, Börje A, Matura M, et al. Studies on the autoxidation and sensitizing capacity of the fragrance chemical linalool, identifying a linalool hydroperoxide. Contact Derm 2002;46(5):267–72.

33. de Groot AC, Schmidt E. Essential oils, part IV: contact allergy. Dermatitis 2016;27(4):170–5.

34. Bråred Christensson J, Andersen KE, Bruze M, et al. Air-oxidized linalool: a frequent cause of fragrance contact allergy. Contact Dermatitis 2012;67(5): 247–59.

35. Bråred Christensson J, Andersen KE, Bruze M, et al. An international multicentre study on the allergenic activity of air-oxidized R-limonene. Contact Dermatitis 2013;68(4):214–23.

36. Schalock PC, Dunnick CA, Nedorost S, et al. American contact dermatitis society core allergen series: 2017 update. Dermatitis 2017;28(2):141–3.

37. Audrain H, Kenward C, Lovell CR, et al. Allergy to oxidized limonene and linalool is frequent in the U.K. Br J Dermatol 2014;171(2):292–7.

38. Ung CY, White JML, White IR, et al. Patch testing with the European baseline series fragrance markers: a 2016 update. Br J Dermatol 2018; 178(3):776–80.

39. Wlodek C, Penfold CM, Bourke JF, et al. Recommendation to test limonene hydroperoxides 0·3% and linalool hydroperoxides 1·0% in the British baseline patch test series. Br J Dermatol 2017;177(6): 1708–15.

40. Yim E, Baquerizo nole KL, Tosti A. Contact dermatitis caused by preservatives. Dermatitis 2014;25(5): 215–31.

41. de Groot AC, White IR, Flyvholm MA, et al. Formaldehyde-releasers in cosmetics: relationship to formaldehyde contact allergy. Part 1. Characterization, frequency and relevance of sensitization, and

frequency of use in cosmetics. Contact Dermatitis 2010;62(1):2–17.

42. Fewing J, Menne T. An update of the risk assessment for methylchloroisothiazolinone/methylisothiazolinone (MCI/MI) with focus on rinse-off products. Contact Dermatitis 2000;41:1–13.

43. Castanedo-tardana MP, Zug KA. Methylisothiazolinone. Dermatitis 2013;24(1):2–6.

44. Wilford JE, de Gannes GC. Methylisothiazolinone contact allergy prevalence in Western Canada: increased detection with 2000 ppm patch test allergen. J Cutan Med Surg 2017;21(3):207–10.

45. Warshaw EM, Belsito DV, Taylor JS, et al. North American contact dermatitis group patch test results: 2011—2012. Dermatitis 2015;26(1):49–59.

46. Cashman AL, Warshaw EM. Parabens: a review of epidemiology, structure, allergenicity, and hormonal properties. Dermatitis 2005;16(2):57–66.

47. Sasseville D, Alfalah M, Lacroix JP. "Parabenoia" debunked, or "who's afraid of parabens?". Dermatitis 2015;26(6):254–9.

48. Castelain F, Castelain M. Parabens: a real hazard or a scare story? Eur J Dermatol 2012;22(6):723–7.

49. Fowler JF. Gold. Am J Contact Dermatitis 2001; 12(1):1–2.

50. Chen JK, Lampel HP. Gold contact allergy: clues and controversies. Dermatitis 2015;26(2):69–77.

51. Goldenberg A, Vassantachart J, Lin EJ, et al. Nickel allergy in adults in the U.S.: 1962 to 2015. Dermatitis 2015;26(5):216–23.

52. Zug KA, Pham AK, Belsito DV, et al. Patch testing in children from 2005 to 2012: results from the North American contact dermatitis group. Dermatitis 2014;25(6):345–55.

53. Warshaw EM, Aschenbeck KA, Dekoven JG, et al. Piercing and metal sensitivity: extended analysis of the North American Contact Dermatitis Group Data, 2007-2014. Dermatitis 2017;28(6):333–41.

54. Fowler JF. Cobalt. Dermatitis 2016;27(1):3–8.

55. Uter W, Gefeller O, Geier J, et al. Contact sensitization to cobalt–multifactorial analysis of risk factors based on long-term data of the Information Network of Departments of Dermatology. Contact Derm 2014;71(6):326–37.

56. Lessmann H, Schnuch A, Geier J, et al. Skin-sensitizing and irritant properties of propylene glycol. Contact Dermatitis 2005;53(5):247–59.

57. Mcgowan MA, Scheman A, Jacob SE. Propylene glycol in contact dermatitis: a systematic review. Dermatitis 2018;29(1):6–12.

58. Jacob SE, Scheman A, Mcgowan MA. Propylene glycol. Dermatitis 2018;29(1):3–5.

59. Warshaw EM, Botto NC, Maibach HI, et al. Positive patch-test reactions to propylene glycol: a retrospective cross-sectional analysis from the North American Contact Dermatitis Group, 1996 to 2006. Dermatitis 2009;20(1):14–20.

60. Wetter DA, Yiannias JA, Prakash AV, et al. Resultsofpatchtestingtopersonal care product allergens in a standard series and a supplemental cosmetic series: an analysis of 945 patients from the Mayo Clinic Contact Dermatitis Group, 2000—2007. J Am Acad Dermatol 2010;63(5):789–98.

61. DeKoven JG, Warshaw EM, Belsito DV, et al. North American Contact Dermatitis Group patch test results 2013-2014. Dermatitis 2017;28(1):33–46.

62. Carlson S, Gipson K, Nedorost S. Relevance of doubtful ("equivocal") late patch-test readings. Dermatitis 2010;21(2):102–8.

63. Deleo VA. p-Phenylenediamine. Dermatitis 2006; 17(2):53–5.

64. Han JH, Lee HJ, Bang CH, et al. P-phenylenediamine hair dye allergy and its clinical characteristics. Ann Dermatol 2018;30(3):316–21.

65. Krasteva M, Bons B, Ryan C, et al. Consumer allergy to oxidative hair coloring products: epidemiologic data in the literature. Dermatitis 2009;20:123–41.

66. de Groot AC. New contact allergens: 2008 to 2015. Dermatitis 2015;26(5):199–215.

67. Karlberg AT, Dooms-Goossens A. Contact allergy to oxidized D-limonene among dermatitis patients. Contact Dermatitis 1997;36(4):201–6.

68. Bennike NH, Zachariae C, Johansen JD. Trends in contact allergy to fragrance mix I in consecutive Danish patients with eczema from 1986 to 2015: a cross-sectional study. Br J Dermatol 2017;176(4): 1035–41.

69. Schalock PC, Crawford G, Nedorost S, et al. Patch testing for evaluation of hypersensitivity to implanted metal devices: a perspective from the American Contact Dermatitis Society. Dermatitis 2016;27(5): 241–7.

70. Contactderm.org (nd). History of Allergen of the Year. Available at: https://www.contactderm.org/i4a/pages/index.cfm?pageid=3467. Accessed July 17, 2018.

Biologics and Psoriasis
The Beat Goes On

Hee J. Kim, MD, Mark G. Lebwohl, MD*

KEYWORDS

• Biologics • Psoriasis • Psoriatic arthritis • Efficacy • Safety • Th17/IL-23 axis

KEY POINTS

- Although there are many biologics that are approved for the treatment of psoriasis, certain biological therapy may be more ideal for psoriasis patients with specific needs.
- High rates of complete clearance of psoriasis have been reported with biologics that target interleukin 17 (IL-17) or IL-23.
- A long-term maintenance of clinical response is observed with the following biologics: ustekinumab, secukinumab, ixekizumab, brodalumab, guselkumab, tildrakizumab, and risankizumab.
- Brodalumab has the earliest onset of efficacy, with less than 2 weeks as the median time taken to achieve at least 50% improvement in psoriasis patients, and is followed shortly thereafter by ixekizumab and secukinumab.
- Newer biological agents that target the IL-23/T helper 17 cell pathways, including ustekinumab, secukinumab, ixekizumab, brodalumab, and guselkumab, do not have boxed warnings indicating high risk of serious infections or malignancies.

INTRODUCTION

Psoriasis is a chronic, immune-mediated, inflammatory skin disease that is prevalent in about 3% of world's population and 3.2% of US adults who are 20 years and older.[1,2] More than 30% of patients with psoriasis develop psoriatic arthritis, which further worsens quality of life and impairs physical function. Because of the chronic nature of psoriasis and psoriatic arthritis, a long-term systemic therapy is often required for optimal treatment and maintenance. In the MAPP (Multinational Assessment of Psoriasis and Psoriatic arthritis) survey, 24.9% and 17.7% of 1005 psoriasis patients in the United States who participated in the survey reported the use of conventional oral systemic and biological therapies, respectively.[2] Over the last 2 decades, the development of biological therapies has revolutionized the management of psoriasis and psoriatic arthritis. Since then, numerous biological agents have been approved for the treatment of psoriasis and psoriatic arthritis, and more are currently in development. Each biological therapy has its own unique mechanism of action, benefits, and side effects as demonstrated by the efficacy and safety data in clinical trials.[3,4] Certain biological therapy may be more suitable for a specific subset of patient population and not all patients may respond well to the initial choice of biological therapy. Therefore, it is imperative to understand major benefits and limitations of each biological therapy. Here, the authors review evidence presented by clinical trials and discuss the ideal choice of biological therapy for psoriasis patients with specific needs.

Disclosure Statement: Dr M.G. Lebwohl is an employee of Mount Sinai, which receives research funds from Abbvie, Amgen, Boehringer Ingelheim, Celgene, Eli Lilly, Janssen/Johnson & Johnson, Kadmon, Medimmune/Astra Zeneca, Novartis, Pfizer and ViDac. Dr M.G. Lebwohl is also a consultant for Allergan, Leopharma, and Promius. Dr H.J. Kim has no financial or commercial conflicting interests to disclose.
Department of Dermatology, Icahn School of Medicine at Mount Sinai, 5 East 98th Street, 5th Floor, PO Box 1048, New York, NY 10029, USA
* Corresponding author.
E-mail address: lebwohl@aol.com

Dermatol Clin 37 (2019) 29–36
https://doi.org/10.1016/j.det.2018.07.004
0733-8635/19/© 2018 Elsevier Inc. All rights reserved.

EFFICACY: PASI-75, PASI-90, AND PASI-100

There are numerous biological therapies that have been approved by the US Food and Drug Administration (FDA) for the treatment of moderate-to-severe plaque psoriasis: tumor necrosis factor alpha (TNFα) inhibitors (etanercept, adalimumab, infliximab), interleukin 12/23 (IL-12/23) inhibitor (ustekinumab), IL-17 inhibitors (secukinumab, ixekizumab, brodalumab), and IL-23 inhibitors (tildrakizumab, guselkumab). In addition to these biologics, there are more currently in development. Data from clinical trials and follow-up evaluations demonstrate that each type of biological therapy varies from one another with regards to efficacy, safety, side effects, and other characteristics.

Tumor Necrosis Factor Alpha Inhibitors

Clinical trials have shown that most patients achieve PASI-75 with most currently available biological agents, which include infliximab, adalimumab, ustekinumab, secukinumab, ixekizumab, brodalumab, guselkumab, and tildrakizumab (**Fig. 1**). More than one-third of patients who receive these biological agents with the exception of etanercept achieved 90% reduction in their PASI scores from baseline. Infliximab is a monoclonal antibody that binds to and inhibits the biological activity of TNFα. There are 3 randomized, double-blind, placebo-controlled studies that

have assessed the safety and efficacy of infliximab in plaque psoriasis. In all 3 studies, 75% to 88% of patients treated with infliximab, 5 mg/kg, achieved PASI-75 at week 10.[5] In one particular study, PASI-75 was maintained until week 24 in 82% of patients and until week 50 in 61% of patients.[6] At week 10, 57% of patients on infliximab achieved at least a PASI-90 and 58% of patients by week 24.[6] Etanercept is a soluble TNF-receptor antagonist, and 2 randomized, double-blind, placebo-controlled studies have evaluated its safety and efficacy in psoriasis. Both studies have demonstrated that PASI-75 at week 12 was attained by 32% of patients treated with subcutaneous etanercept, 25 mg, twice weekly and by 46% to 47% of patients treated with etanercept, 50 mg, twice weekly.[7] With 50 mg twice weekly dosing, 49% of patients maintained PASI-75 at week 24, compared with 3% in the placebo group.[8] Adalimumab is a fully human monoclonal antibody that binds to and inhibits the activity of human TNF. Two randomized, double-blind, placebo-controlled trials have been conducted. At week 16, 71% to 78% of patients randomized to adalimumab, 40 mg, every other week achieved 75% reduction in their PASI scores from baseline, compared with 7% to 19% in the placebo group.[9] In a multicenter phase III study, 45% and 20% of patients treated with adalimumab achieved PASI-90 and PASI-100 at week 16, respectively.[10]

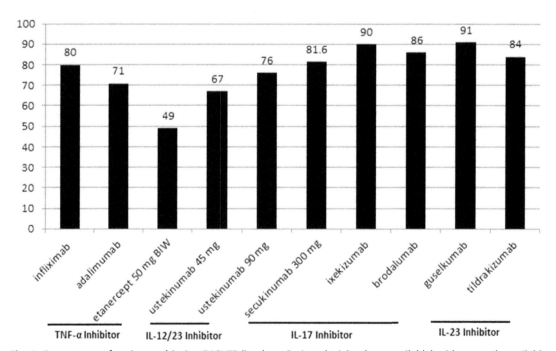

Fig. 1. Percentages of patients achieving PASI-75 (in phase 3 pivotal trials where available) with currently available biological agents (infliximab, etanercept, adalimumab, ustekinumab, secukinumab, ixekizumab, brodalumab, guselkumab, and tildrakizumab) at primary endpoint (week 10–16).

Interleukin-12/23, Interleukin-17, and Interleukin-23 Inhibitors

Ustekinumab is a human monoclonal antibody that binds to the p40 subunit of both IL-12 and 23. Two randomized, double-blind, placebo-controlled trials (PHOENIX1 and PHOENIX2) have assessed the efficacy and safety of ustekinumab in patients with plaque psoriasis.[11–13] In both studies, PASI-75 was achieved at week 12 by 67% and 66% to 76% of patients who received ustekinumab, 45 mg, and ustekinumab, 90 mg, every 12 weeks, respectively, compared with 3% to 4% of patients in the placebo group.[12,13] PASI-90 was achieved at week 12 by 36.7% to 42.3% and 41.6% to 50.9% of patients in the ustekinumab, 45 mg, and ustekinumab, 90 mg, group, respectively. By week 28, the percentages of patients with PASI-90 were 44.8% to 49.2% and 54.3% to 55.6%, respectively for the ustekinumab, 45 mg, and ustekinumab, 90 mg, group.[12,13] Secukinumab is a fully human monoclonal antibody that neutralizes IL-17A. There are 4 randomized, double-blind, placebo-controlled, phase III trials that have examined the safety and efficacy of secukinumab in plaque psoriasis subjects.[14] In all 4 trials, high percentage of patients in the secukinumab group reached PASI-75 at week 12: 75% to 87% of subjects who received secukinumab, 300 mg, every 4 weeks and 67% to 71% of subjects who received secukinumab, 150 mg, every 4 weeks, compared with 0% to 5% of those who received placebo.[14–16] In a global, multicenter, phase III study (ERASURE), 59.2% of subjects who received secukinumab, 300 mg, 39.1% of subjects who received secukinumab, 150 mg, and 2.4% of subjects on placebo achieved PASI-90 at week 12.[16] In a phase III comparative study of secukinumab versus etanercept, 54.2% of patients in the secukinumab, 300 mg, group and 41.9% of patients in the 150 mg group reached PASI-90 at week 12, compared with 20.7% in the etanercept group and 1.5% in the placebo group.[15]

Three of the newest IL-17 and IL-23 inhibitors approved for psoriasis have demonstrated superior efficacy in skin clearance with more than one-third of subjects achieving 100% improvement from baseline PASI after 12 to 16 weeks of biological exposure. These biological agents include ixekizumab, brodalumab, and guselkumab. Ixekizumab is a monoclonal antibody that targets IL-17A. Three phase III studies (UNCOVER-1, 2, 3) have evaluated its efficacy and safety in the treatment of psoriatic plaques.[17] In all 3 studies, 87% to 90% of subjects who received ixekizumab, 80 mg, every 2 weeks achieved PASI-75, 68% to 71% of

subjects achieved PASI-90, and 35% to 40% of subjects achieved PASI-100 at week 12.[18,19] Brodalumab is a monoclonal antibody that blocks the activity of IL-17 receptor A. Three multicenter, randomized, double-blind, phase III studies have assessed the safety and efficacy of brodalumab in subjects with moderate-to-severe plaque psoriasis.[20] All 3 studies showed excellent results: at week 12, 83% to 86% of patients randomized to receive brodalumab, 210 mg, every 2 weeks achieved PASI-75 and 37% to 44% of patients achieved PASI-100.[21] Guselkumab is a human monoclonal antibody that binds to and inhibits IL-23. Two phase III studies have assessed the efficacy and safety of guselkumab (VOYAGE1, VOYAGE2).[22] In both VOYAGE1 and VOYAGE2, 83% to 91% of subjects who received guselkumab, 100 mg, every 8 weeks reached PASI-75 at week 16 and 64% to 73% of subjects reached PASI-90 at week 16.[22] VOYAGE2 study showed that 34.1% of subjects in the guselkumab group achieved PASI-100 at week 16 and the percentage of patients with PASI-100 increased up to 44.2% at week 24.[23]

MAINTENANCE OF DISEASE CONTROL

Given the chronic course of disease, psoriasis requires an effective long-term treatment with high durability of disease control. Thus, it is important to understand the maintenance of clinical response associated with each biological therapy. The following biological therapies have demonstrated long-term maintenance of effective clinical response: ustekinumab, secukinumab, ixekizumab, brodalumab, guselkumab, tildrakizumab, and risankizumab.

Interleukin-12/23 Inhibitor

In PHOENIX1 and PHOENIX2, patients receiving maintenance therapy of either ustekinumab, 45 mg, or ustekinumab, 90 mg, sustained PASI-50, PASI-75, or PASI-90 responses up to either 52 or 76 weeks.[12,13] At week 244, PASI-75 was maintained by 76.5% and 78.6% of patients randomized to ustekinumab, 45 mg, and ustekinumab, 90 mg, respectively. PASI-90 was maintained by 50.0% and 55.5% of those who received ustekinumab, 45 mg, and ustekinumab, 90 mg, respectively.[24]

Interleukin-17 Inhibitors

Follow-up 5-year data have demonstrated that patients treated with fixed-dose maintenance regimen of secukinumab, 300 mg, sustained improvement from baseline PASI score through

5 years.[25] Among patients treated with secukinumab, 300 mg, at fixed-dose interval, 88.9% of patients achieved PASI-75, 68.5% achieved PASI-90%, and 43.8% achieved PASI-100 at year 1; improvement from baseline PASI score was well-sustained up to year 5 with 88.5%, 66.4%, and 41% of patients maintaining PASI-75, PASI-90, and PASI-100, respectively.[25] Integrated data analysis from 3 phase III studies for ixekizumab (UNCOVER-1, 2, 3) has exhibited that more than 60% of patients who initially had no response or partial response at week 12 were able to achieve PASI-50 response by week 20, and more than 35% were able to achieve PASI-75 response.[26] In UNCOVER-3, patients on ixekizumab maintained high response rates through 108 weeks with more than 70% of patients preserving PASI-90 and more than 50% of patients preserving PASI-100 at week 108.[19] Extension and follow-up study results have shown that brodalumab, 210 mg, administered every 2 weeks is effective in maintaining high PASI responses (PASI-75, 90, 100) through 5 years. At week 12, 95%, 85%, and 63% of patients on brodalumab achieved PASI-75, 90, and 100, respectively. These PASI responses were sustained through week 120 as observed by 86%, 70%, and 51% of patients achieving PASI-75, 90, and 100, respectively.[27]

Interleukin-23 Inhibitors

In VOYAGE1 and VOYAGE2 open-label extension studies, subjects on guselkumab maintained high rates of improvement in baseline PASI through 2 years.[28,29] Approximately 78.9% to 80.1% of patients achieved at least 90% improvement in baseline PASI score by week 52, and this response was maintained at week 100 by 81.1% to 82.3% of patients. Also, 46.6% to 50.5% of patients had complete clearance of psoriasis (PASI-100) at week 52, and this response was maintained at week 100 by 49% to 55.1% of patients.[29] In open-label extension studies (reSURFACE1, reSURFACE2) evaluating the efficacy of tildrakizumab, 100 mg, given every 12 weeks, patients on tildrakizumab maintained same level of efficacy through week 64.[30] At week 64, 84% of patients on tildrakizumab achieved PASI-75, 52% achieved PASI-90, and 22% achieved PASI-100.[30]

EARLY ONSET OF EFFICACY

On average, biological therapies are able to produce effective clinical outcome within 2 to 11 weeks.[31] There are 3 biological agents that are notable for early onset of efficacy as measured by the median time taken to achieve 50% improvement in baseline PASI scores: brodalumab, ixekizumab, and secukinumab (Fig. 2). Brodalumab has the most rapid onset of action in the treatment of psoriasis. A study has demonstrated that the median time to achieve at least 50% improvement in PASI score from baseline with brodalumab was less than 2 weeks and the time taken to achieve at least 75% improvement in PASI score was 4 weeks.[21] Ixekizumab had similar results with 2.1 weeks as the median time to onset of

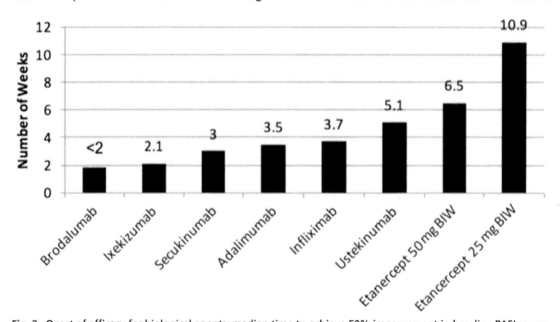

Fig. 2. Onset of efficacy for biological agents: median time to achieve 50% improvement in baseline PASI scores. Comparative biologics are shown as weighted means based on individual study published results.

PASI-50, compared with 8.1 weeks for etanercept.[18,19] For secukinumab, the onset of efficacy differed depending on the dose used. The median time to achieve at least 50% improvement in baseline PASI score was 3 weeks with the higher dose of secukinumab (300 mg) and 3.9 weeks with the lower dose (150 mg).[15] The median time required to achieve 50% reduction in baseline PASI for other biologics are as follows: 3.5 weeks for adalimumab, 3.7 weeks for infliximab, 5.1 weeks for low-dose ustekinumab, 6.5 weeks for high-dose etanercept, and 10.9 weeks for low-dose etanercept.[31]

SAFETY

In addition to superior efficacy, biological agents have shown good safety profiles compared with conventional systemic agents such as methotrexate. Boxed warnings associated with methotrexate include fetal death/congenital anomalies, bone marrow suppression, gastrointestinal toxicity with concomitant nonsteroidal antiinflammatory drug use, hepatotoxicity, cirrhosis, pulmonary toxicity, malignant lymphomas, bone marrow suppression, and infections.[32–34] According to guidelines, patients on methotrexate require regular monitoring of liver enzymes and blood counts due to toxic effects of methotrexate on liver and bone marrow.

Tumor Necrosis Factor Inhibitors

Anti-TNF drugs used for the treatment of psoriasis (infliximab, etanercept, and adalimumab) have shown to be associated with higher risk of serious infections, tuberculosis, and malignancies such as lymphoma. Guidelines recommend monitoring for active tuberculosis during treatment with anti-TNFs regardless of negative result for latent TB initially.[35,36] A study evaluating long-term safety and efficacy of etanercept therapy demonstrated relatively constant rate of safety profile with up to 10 years of etanercept therapy exposure.[37] In a safety analysis of more than 12 years of adalimumab exposure in 23,458 patients from global clinical trials in rheumatoid arthritis (RA), juvenile idiopathic arthritis, ankylosing spondylitis, psoriatic arthritis, psoriasis, and Crohn's disease, infections were found to be the most frequently reported serious adverse events as expected from previously reported trials. Opportunistic infections, serious demyelinating disorders, and congestive heart failure were rarely reported, and the incidence of malignancy was consistent with previously reported rates.[38]

Some studies have demonstrated beneficial effects of anti-TNF use. The association between anti-TNF treatments and reduced mortality risk has been demonstrated in a study that compared morality rates in patients with RA treated with TNF inhibitors and those of a standard RA population. Mortality rates were 51 deaths per 3177 patient-years among patients with RA treated with anti-TNF and 137 deaths per 3900 patient-years among those not treated.[39] Anti-TNF drugs have also been reported to lower the risk of first cardiovascular events, cardiovascular disease, and myocardial infarction.[40–42]

Newer Biologics: Interleukin-12/23, Interleukin-17, and Interleukin-23 Inhibitors

Newer biological agents that target the IL-23/Th17 pathways, including ustekinumab, secukinumab, ixekizumab, brodalumab, and guselkumab, offer superior efficacy and safety compared with conventional systemic therapies and TNFα inhibitors. They do not have boxed warnings indicating high risk of serious infections and malignancies, but they do have common adverse events that have been reported in clinical trials that are limited to mild upper respiratory tract infections, nasopharyngitis, and headache.[43] Studies have reported potential increased risk of mucocutaneous candidiasis with IL-17 inhibitors. A study comparing safety profiles of secukinumab and etanercept has demonstrated that secukinumab-treated patients had higher frequency of mild-to-moderate, mucocutaneous *Candida* infections compared with those treated with either etanercept or placebo.[44–46] Unlike TNF inhibitors, occurrences of serious infections, reactivation of latent tuberculosis or hepatitis B, lymphoma, or other malignancies have not been reported with long-term use of IL-17 inhibitors.[44] Brodalumab (SILIQ) has a black box warning regarding suicidal ideation or behavior, and it is only available through the SILIQ REMS (Risk Evaluation Mitigation Safety) program. However, studies have demonstrated that there is lack of evidence to establish causality between brodalumab and increased risk of suicidal ideation or behavior. In a group of patients treated with brodalumab, the incidence of suicidal attempts or completed suicides did not increase with time.[47]

SPECIAL POPULATION WITH SPECIFIC NEEDS
Obesity: Adjust for Weight

Most biological therapies are administered in fixed dose regimens with the exception of infliximab and ustekinumab, which are adjusted based on body weight. Other biologics can be dose-adjusted such as secukinumab and certolizumab. Studies have reported that patients with body weight greater than 100 kg, who make up almost 25% to 30% of patients in clinical trials, have reduced clinical response to fixed-dose biological therapies.[48] A significant improvement in the efficacy of biological therapy in psoriasis treatment has been reported in obese patients who underwent body weight reduction by dietary control.[49] A weight-dependent PASI response has been observed in a study evaluating 2 different doses of ustekinumab in psoriasis treatment. In subjects with weight 100 kg or less, 73% to 74% of patients in the ustekinumab, 45 mg, group and 65% to 78% of patients in the ustekinumab, 90 mg, group reached PASI-75 response at week 12. In subjects with weight greater than 100 kg, 49% to 54% of patients who received ustekinumab, 45 mg, achieved PASI-75 at week 12, compared with 68% to 71% of patients who received ustekinumab, 90 mg.[12,13] Novel biological agents that target the IL-23/Th17 pathways have been shown to be very effective regardless of body weight, and these include secukinumab, ixekizumab, brodalumab, guselkumab, tildrakizumab, risankizumab, and mirikizumab.

Concomitant Psoriatic Arthritis

For patients with psoriasis and concomitant psoriatic arthritis, TNF blockers and anti-IL-17 drugs are most effective. According to PSUMMIT-1 and PSUMMIT-2 studies, both ustekinumab, 45 mg, and ustekinumab, 90 mg, treatments have been shown to reduce radiographic progression of joint damage in patients with active psoriatic arthritis although not as much as TNF blockers.[50] In the extension study for ixekizumab, radiographic progression of joint damage was minimal with either 40 mg every 2 week or every 4 week regimen, and the extent of reduction in sharp scores was comparable to the reduction with adalimumab.[51]

Safety in Pregnancy

There is limited data on the safety of biological agents in pregnancy. Various cases of safe use of biological agents in pregnancy have been reported; however, some adverse pregnancy outcomes including congenital malformation without clear pattern have been reported as well.[52] Certolizumab pegol (CZP) is the only Fc-free, anti-TNF biological agent that does not bind to the neonatal Fc receptor for immunoglobulin G and subsequently minimizes potential transfer through the placenta and breast milk from mother to infant. CZP was recently approved by FDA for treatment of psoriasis in May 2018.[53]

Fewer Injections

As a chronic disease, psoriasis requires a lifelong maintenance of disease control. Newer biological agents with a fewer number of required injections per year are being developed to meet the needs of psoriasis patients. The following biologics are administered every 2 to 3 months: ustekinumab, tildrakizumab, guselkumab, and risankizumab.[11,22,54]

REFERENCES

1. Rachakonda TD, Schupp CW, Armstrong AW. Psoriasis prevalence among adults in the United States. J Am Acad Dermatol 2014;70(3):512–6.
2. Lebwohl MG, Kavanaugh A, Armstrong AW, et al. US perspectives in the management of psoriasis and psoriatic arthritis: patient and physician results from the population-based multinational assessment of psoriasis and psoriatic arthritis (MAPP) survey. Am J Clin Dermatol 2016;17(1):87–97.
3. Amin M, No DJ, Egeberg A, et al. Choosing first-line biologic treatment for moderate-to-severe psoriasis: what does the evidence say? Am J Clin Dermatol 2018;19(1):1–13.
4. Menter A, Gottlieb A, Feldman SR, et al. Guidelines of care for the management of psoriasis and psoriatic arthritis: section 1. Overview of psoriasis and guidelines of care for the treatment of psoriasis with biologics. J Am Acad Dermatol 2008;58(5): 826–50.
5. Remicade® (infliximab) [package insert]. Horsham, PA: Janssen Biotech, Inc.; 1998.
6. Reich K, Nestle FO, Papp K, et al. Infliximab induction and maintenance therapy for moderate-to-severe psoriasis: a phase III, multicentre, double-blind trial. Lancet 2005;366(9494): 1367–74.
7. Enbrel® (etanercept) [package insert]. Thousand Oaks, CA: Immunex Corporation; 1998.
8. Papp KA, Tyring S, Lahfa M, et al. A global phase III randomized controlled trial of etanercept in psoriasis: safety, efficacy, and effect of dose reduction. Br J Dermatol 2005;152(6):1304–12.
9. HUMIRA® (adalimumab) [package insert]. North Chicago, IL: Abbott Laboratories; 2002.
10. Menter A, Tyring SK, Gordon K, et al. Adalimumab therapy for moderate to severe psoriasis: a randomized, controlled phase III trial. J Am Acad Dermatol 2008;58(1):106–15.
11. STELARA® (ustekinumab) [package insert]. Horsham, PA: Janssen Biotech, Inc.; 2009.
12. Leonardi CL, Kimball AB, Papp KA, et al. Efficacy and safety of ustekinumab, a human interleukin-12/23 monoclonal antibody, in patients with psoriasis: 76-week results from a randomised, double-blind, placebo-controlled trial (PHOENIX 1). Lancet 2008; 371(9625):1665–74.
13. Papp KA, Langley RG, Lebwohl M, et al. Efficacy and safety of ustekinumab, a human interleukin-12/

23 monoclonal antibody, in patients with psoriasis: 52-week results from a randomised, double-blind, placebo-controlled trial (PHOENIX 2). Lancet 2008; 371(9625):1675–84.

14. COSENTYX® (secukinumab) [package insert]. East Hanover, NJ: Novartis Pharmaceuticals Corporation; 2015.

15. Langley RG, Elewski BE, Lebwohl M, et al. Secukinumab in plaque psoriasis–results of two phase 3 trials. N Engl J Med 2014;371(4):326–38.

16. Ohtsuki M, Morita A, Abe M, et al. Secukinumab efficacy and safety in Japanese patients with moderate-to-severe plaque psoriasis: subanalysis from ERASURE, a randomized, placebo-controlled, phase 3 study. J Dermatol 2014;41(12):1039–46.

17. TALTZ (ixekizumab) [package insert]. Indianapolis, IN: Eli Lilly and Company; 2016.

18. Papp KA, Leonardi CL, Blauvelt A, et al. Ixekizumab treatment for psoriasis: integrated efficacy analysis of three double-blinded, controlled studies (UNCOVER-1, UNCOVER-2, UNCOVER-3). Br J Dermatol 2018;178(3):674–81.

19. Blauvelt A, Gooderham M, Iversen L, et al. Efficacy and safety of ixekizumab for the treatment of moderate-to-severe plaque psoriasis: results through 108 weeks of a randomized, controlled phase 3 clinical trial (UNCOVER-3). J Am Acad Dermatol 2017;77(5):855–62.

20. SILIQ™ (brodalumab) [package insert]. Bridgewater, NJ: Valeant Pharmaceuticals North America LLC; 2017.

21. Lebwohl M, Strober B, Menter A, et al. Phase 3 studies comparing brodalumab with ustekinumab in psoriasis. N Engl J Med 2015;373(14):1318–28.

22. Tremfya™ (guselkumab) [package insert]. Horsham, PA: Janssen Biotech, Inc.; 2017.

23. Reich K, Armstrong AW, Foley P, et al. Efficacy and safety of guselkumab, an anti-interleukin-23 monoclonal antibody, compared with adalimumab for the treatment of patients with moderate to severe psoriasis with randomized withdrawal and retreatment: Results from the phase III, double-blind, placebo- and active comparator-controlled VOYAGE 2 trial. J Am Acad Dermatol 2017;76(3): 418–31.

24. Langley RG, Lebwohl M, Krueger GG, et al. Long-term efficacy and safety of ustekinumab, with and without dosing adjustment, in patients with moderate-to-severe psoriasis: results from the PHOENIX 2 study through 5 years of follow-up. Br J Dermatol 2015;172(5):1371–83.

25. Bissonnette R, Luger T, Thaci D, et al. Secukinumab demonstrates high sustained efficacy and a favourable safety profile in patients with moderate-to-severe psoriasis through 5 years of treatment (SCULPTURE Extension Study). J Eur Acad Dermatol Venereol 2018. [Epub ahead of print].

26. Kemeny L, Berggren L, Dossenbach M, et al. Efficacy and safety of ixekizumab in patients with plaque psoriasis across different degrees of disease severity: results from UNCOVER-2 and UNCOVER-3. J Dermatolog Treat 2018;1–27. [Epub ahead of print].

27. Papp K, Leonardi C, Menter A, et al. Safety and efficacy of brodalumab for psoriasis after 120 weeks of treatment. J Am Acad Dermatol 2014;71(6):1183–90.e3.

28. Blauvelt A, Papp KA, Griffiths CE, et al. Efficacy and safety of guselkumab, an anti-interleukin-23 monoclonal antibody, compared with adalimumab for the continuous treatment of patients with moderate to severe psoriasis: results from the phase III, double-blinded, placebo- and active comparator-controlled VOYAGE 1 trial. J Am Acad Dermatol 2017;76(3):405–17.

29. Griffiths CE, Papp KA, et al. 26th European academy of dermatology and venereology congress (EADV 2017) 13–17 September, 2017; Geneva, Switzerland; D3T01.1l.

30. Reich K, Papp KA, Blauvelt A, et al. Tildrakizumab versus placebo or etanercept for chronic plaque psoriasis (reSURFACE 1 and reSURFACE 2): results from two randomised controlled, phase 3 trials. Lancet 2017;390(10091):276–88.

31. Papp KA, Lebwohl MG. Onset of action of biologics in patients with moderate-to-severe psoriasis. J Drugs Dermatol 2017;17(3):247–50.

32. Schmitt J, Rosumeck S, Thomaschewski G, et al. Efficacy and safety of systemic treatments for moderate-to-severe psoriasis: meta-analysis of randomized controlled trials. Br J Dermatol 2014; 170(2):274–303.

33. Visser K, van der Heijde DM. Risk and management of liver toxicity during methotrexate treatment in rheumatoid and psoriatic arthritis: a systematic review of the literature. Clin Exp Rheumatol 2009; 27(6):1017–25.

34. Menter A, Korman NJ, Elmets CA, et al. Guidelines of care for the management of psoriasis and psoriatic arthritis: section 4. Guidelines of care for the management and treatment of psoriasis with traditional systemic agents. J Am Acad Dermatol 2009; 61(3):451–85.

35. Garcia-Doval I, Cohen AD, Cazzaniga S, et al. Risk of serious infections, cutaneous bacterial infections, and granulomatous infections in patients with psoriasis treated with anti-tumor necrosis factor agents versus classic therapies: prospective meta-analysis of Psonet registries. J Am Acad Dermatol 2017;76(2):299–308.e16.

36. Kamata M, Tada Y. Safety of biologics in psoriasis. J Dermatol 2018;45(3):279–86.

37. Weinblatt ME, Bathon JM, Kremer JM, et al. Safety and efficacy of etanercept beyond 10 years of therapy in North American patients with early and long-standing rheumatoid arthritis. Arthritis Care Res 2011;63(3):373–82.

38. Burmester GR, Panaccione R, Gordon KB, et al. Adalimumab: long-term safety in 23 458 patients from global clinical trials in rheumatoid arthritis, juvenile idiopathic arthritis, ankylosing spondylitis, psoriatic arthritis, psoriasis and Crohn's disease. Ann Rheum Dis 2013;72(4):517–24.

39. Jacobsson LT, Turesson C, Nilsson JA, et al. Treatment with TNF blockers and mortality risk in patients with rheumatoid arthritis. Ann Rheum Dis 2007; 66(5):670–5.

40. Jacobsson LT, Turesson C, Gulfe A, et al. Treatment with tumor necrosis factor blockers is associated with a lower incidence of first cardiovascular events in patients with rheumatoid arthritis. J Rheumatol 2005;32(7):1213–8.

41. Dixon WG, Watson KD, Lunt M, et al. Reduction in the incidence of myocardial infarction in patients with rheumatoid arthritis who respond to anti-tumor necrosis factor alpha therapy: results from the British Society for Rheumatology Biologics Register. Arthritis Rheum 2007;56(9):2905–12.

42. Wu JJ, Poon KY, Channual JC, et al. Association between tumor necrosis factor inhibitor therapy and myocardial infarction risk in patients with psoriasis. Arch Dermatol 2012;148(11):1244–50.

43. Dong J, Goldenberg G. New biologics in psoriasis: an update on IL-23 and IL-17 inhibitors. Cutis 2017;99(2):123–7.

44. Blauvelt A. Safety of secukinumab in the treatment of psoriasis. Expert Opin Drug Saf 2016;15(10):1413–20.

45. Puel A, Cypowyj S, Marodi L, et al. Inborn errors of human IL-17 immunity underlie chronic mucocutaneous candidiasis. Curr Opin Allergy Clin Immunol 2012;12(6):616–22.

46. Cypowyj S, Picard C, Marodi L, et al. Immunity to infection in IL-17-deficient mice and humans. Eur J Immunol 2012;42(9):2246–54.

47. Lebwohl MG, Papp KA, Marangell LB, et al. Psychiatric adverse events during treatment with brodalumab: analysis of psoriasis clinical trials. J Am Acad Dermatol 2018; 78(1):81–9.e5.

48. Puig L. Obesity and psoriasis: body weight and body mass index influence the response to biological treatment. J Eur Acad Dermatol Venereol 2011; 25(9):1007–11.

49. Al-Mutairi N, Nour T. The effect of weight reduction on treatment outcomes in obese patients with psoriasis on biologic therapy: a randomized controlled prospective trial. Expert Opin Biol Ther 2014;14(6):749–56.

50. Kavanaugh A, Ritchlin C, Rahman P, et al. Ustekinumab, an anti-IL-12/23 p40 monoclonal antibody, inhibits radiographic progression in patients with active psoriatic arthritis: results of an integrated analysis of radiographic data from the phase 3, multicentre, randomised, double-blind, placebo-controlled PSUMMIT-1 and PSUMMIT-2 trials. Ann Rheum Dis 2014;73(6):1000–6.

51. van der Heijde D, Gladman DD, Kishimoto M, et al. Efficacy and safety of ixekizumab in patients with active psoriatic arthritis: 52-week results from a phase III study (SPIRIT-P1). J Rheumatol 2018; 45(3):367–77.

52. Murase JE, Heller MM, Butler DC. Safety of dermatologic medications in pregnancy and lactation: part I. Pregnancy. J Am Acad Dermatol 2014;70(3):401.e1-14 [quiz: 415].

53. CIMZIA (certolizumab pegol) [package insert]. Smyrna, GA: UCB, Inc.; 2008.

54. ILUMYA™ (tildrakizumab-asmn) [pacakge insert]. Whitehouse station, NJ: Merck & Co., Inc.; 2018.

Connective Tissue Disease
Current Concepts

Anthony P. Fernandez, MD, PhD

KEYWORDS

- Connective tissue disease • Dermatomyositis • Cutaneous lupus erythematosus • Morphea
- Cutaneous vasculitis

KEY POINTS

- Classification criteria for dermatomyositis that includes amyopathic patients has recently been published and several medications effective for patients with refractory cutaneous dermatomyositis have been described.
- Progress in objectively defining cutaneous lupus erythematosus, updates in pathogenesis, and studies optimizing antimalarial use in patients with cutaneous lupus erythematosus have occurred in recent years.
- There have been updates in clinical features of patients with morphea, in addition to the identification of several potential biomarkers of disease activity and novel treatments.
- Clarification of categories applicable to skin vasculitis have recently been described and clinical studies that aim to better understand pathogenesis and identify effective treatments are ongoing.

INTRODUCTION

Connective tissue diseases can affect numerous organ systems and often prominently affect the skin. Thus, dermatologists frequently play an important role in the diagnosis and management of these conditions. Herein is an update of our understanding of various aspects of common connective tissue diseases, with many contributions resulting from research performed by dermatologists with expertise in these diseases.

DERMATOMYOSITIS

Dermatomyositis (DM) is an autoimmune disease that most commonly affects the skin and muscles.

A number of important updates concerning DM have occurred in recent years that are particularly pertinent to dermatologists who treat these patients. Arguably, the most important is the release of updated idiopathic inflammatory myopathy (IIM) classification guidelines by the European League Against Rheumatism/American College of Rheumatology (EULAR/ACR) that help accurately distinguish DM from other IIMs.[1] Unlike the classic criteria published by Bohan and Peter,[2,3] the new EULAR/ACR classification criteria included patients with clinically amyopathic DM (CADM), as well as comparators with other dermatologic disease, in their study population. The EULAR/ACR classification criteria take into account several cutaneous manifestations of DM, including

Disclosure Statement: Dr A.P. Fernandez is a Principal Investigator and receives funding from Mallinckrodt (Efficacy and Safety of H.P. Acthar gel for the treatment of refractory cutaneous manifestations of dermatomyositis; ClinicalTrials.gov identifier NCT02245841) and Pfizer (A Phase 2a, Double-blind, Randomized, Placebo-controlled Study To Evaluate The Efficacy, Safety, And Tolerability Of Pf-06823859 In Adult Subjects With Dermatomyositis; ClinicalTrials.gov identifier NCT03181893) for dermatomyositis research and is a consultant for Celgene. He also is an investigator for the ARAMIS (ClinicalTrials.gov identifier NCT02939573) and CUTIS (ClinicalTrials.gov identifier NCT03004326) studies.
Departments of Dermatology and Pathology, Cleveland Clinic Lerner College of Medicine, 9500 Euclid Avenue A61, Cleveland, OH 44195, USA
E-mail address: fernana6@ccf.org

Dermatol Clin 37 (2019) 37–48
https://doi.org/10.1016/j.det.2018.07.006
0733-8635/19/© 2018 Elsevier Inc. All rights reserved.

Gottron's papules, Gottron's sign, and heliotrope rash. By using the EULAR/ACR classification criteria, patients with these pathognomonic skin manifestations of juvenile and adult DM were accurately classified without including muscle biopsy data. For DM patients without muscle involvement, the new criteria recommend a skin biopsy is performed to further support a DM diagnosis.

The EULAR/ACR idiopathic inflammatory myopathy classification criteria represent a tremendous step forward for dermatologists who see patients with DM for several reasons. Not only are specific skin manifestations recognized as important features of DM that can be used for accurate classification, but patients with CADM are now formally accepted as having DM and can theoretically qualify for clinical trials that may lead to improved treatment options for this subset of patients. With that being said, there is still room for improvement in DM classification criteria from a dermatologic standpoint. In a recently published retrospective study of a single-center DM cohort, 26.3% of patients with CADM still would not meet the suggested 55% minimum probability cutoff to be classified as having DM based on the EULAR/ACR criteria.[4] The authors of this study propose inclusion of other cutaneous-specific criteria, such as skin biopsy findings, may improve classification criteria to include a higher percentage of CADM patients.

Control of cutaneous DM disease activity is important for numerous reasons. Cutaneous DM disease is associated with physical symptoms (pain, pruritus), infection risk, and adverse psychological effects, all of which contribute to a significant negative impact on patients' quality of life.[5,6] Furthermore, persistent cutaneous DM can lead to permanent damage in the form of scarring, calcinosis, decreased range of motion, and/or lipoatrophy.

It has long been suspected by some that cutaneous DM manifestations often persist despite aggressive treatment and myositis resolution. Studies in patients with juvenile DM have found up to 60% have persistent cutaneous disease and the percentage with persistent cutaneous disease is often more than double the percentage with persistent myositis.[7–9] However, studies in adults with DM suggesting persistent cutaneous disease activity have been lacking. Recently, a cohort of adult DM patients was prospectively studied to determine the percentage who achieved clinical remission of their cutaneous disease over a 3-year follow-up period.[10] The authors found only 28 of 74 patients (38%) achieved clinical remission over 3 years despite aggressive

systemic therapy treatment regimens. Thus, a significant percentage of DM adult patients, too, are refractory to standard-of-care therapies. Overall, these data reveal that DM cutaneous disease, in general, can often be refractory to treatment and support there is an unmet need for development of more effective cutaneous DM treatments.

Luckily, during the past few years research has identified several medications with promising efficacy in treating refractory cutaneous DM that may eventually be welcome additions to routine therapy armamentariums. Two Janus kinase inhibitors, ruxolitinib and tofacitinib, have recently been reported to effectively treat DM patients, all of whom had refractory cutaneous disease despite exposure to between 4 and 9 systemic medications.[11,12] Although 3 patients were reported to respond well to tofacitinib 5 to 10 mg twice daily in one of the reports, the authors now have accumulated a cohort of at least 9 patients with refractory cutaneous DM who are responding well to tofacitinib (Dr Ruth Ann Vleugals, MD, as presented at the 4th International Cutaneous Lupus and Dermatomyositis meeting; Orlando, FL; personal communication, 2018).

Adrenocorticotropic hormone gel (repository corticotropin hormone [RCI]) has been approved by the US Food and Drug Administration to treat DM and other immune-mediated diseases since 1952. However, there has been a paucity of data concerning efficacy and safety of this treatment for DM. A recent open-label trial reported RCI treatment was both safe and efficacious for DM.[13] Although the focus was on control of myositis, the authors did report 4 of the 5 DM patients (80%) with significant skin disease responded positively to RCI treatment, showing an 88% (83.3%–100%) improvement in cutaneous visual analog scale score. Our group is conducting an open-label study focusing on safety and efficacy of RCI for refractory cutaneous DM disease.[14] Interim results for 9 patients enrolled thus far are similar to what was seen by Aggarwal and colleagues.[13] Improvement in skin disease activity as measured by the Cutaneous Dermatomyositis Activity and Severity Index (CDASI) has been seen in 7 of the 9 patients 3 months after initiating RCI, and in all 7 patients who have so far completed 6 months of the study (Fig. 1). Additionally, there has been improvement in numerous patient-reported outcomes, including the Global Itch Score and Dermatology Life Quality Index scores.

Another promising medication for cutaneous DM is lenabasum (anabasum), a synthetic, oral, preferential cannabinoid 2 receptor agonist. Lenabasum is nonimmunosuppressive and results in reduction

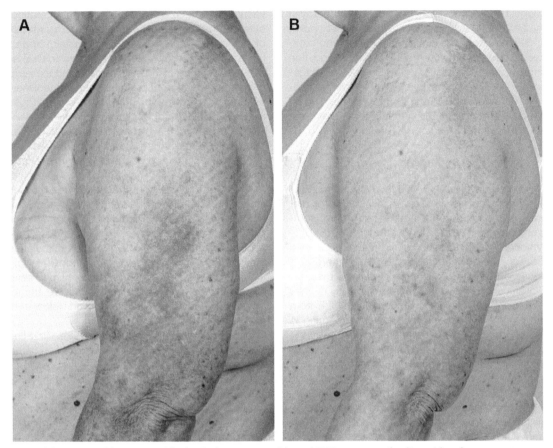

Fig. 1. (*A*) 61-year-old woman with classic dermatomyositis and TIF1-γ autoantibodies with refractory cutaneous disease activity after failing 6 systemic treatments, including multidrug regimens. (*B*) There is significant improvement in her rash 3 months after treatment with repository corticotropin gel (80 U twice weekly) in the setting of an open-label clinical trial (ClinicalTrials.gov identifier NCT02245841). (*From* Fernandez A. Efficacy and Safety of H.P. Acthar Gel for the Treatment of Refractory Cutaneous Manifestations of Dermatomyositis (Acthar Gel) - ClinicalTrials.gov identifier: NCT02245841. Available at: https://clinicaltrials.gov/ct2/show/NCT02245841; with permission.)

of peripheral blood mononuclear cell cytokine production in DM patients, in addition to inducing resolution of innate immune responses.[15] In a double-blind, randomized, placebo-controlled phase II trial, lenabasum provided statistically significant improvement in CDASI activity scores and other secondary efficacy outcomes and displayed excellent tolerability.[16] An open-label extension of this trial supports lenabasum has persistent efficacy, safety and tolerability in patients with refractory skin-predominant DM.[17]

One of the most potentially critical findings concerning cutaneous DM relates to the associated inflammatory cytokine profile. DM is known to be a type I interferon (IFN)-mediated disease, and theoretically could be primarily driven by IFN-α, IFN-β, or other type I IFNs. However, it has recently been shown IFN-β, not

IFN-α, correlates best with DM cutaneous disease activity.[18–20] These findings obviously have potential treatment implications. Sifalimumab, a monoclonal antibody against IFN-α, has been studied as a DM treatment, but its development has been terminated by MedImmune, LLC.[21,22] Thus, it may be that targeting IFN-β is a more effective strategy for controlling DM than targeting IFN- α. Clinical investigations concerning this strategy may be available in the near future.

Finally, dermatologists know well that scalp pruritus can be particularly disturbing for DM patients and refractory to treatment. A recent study revealed the mean epidermal nerve fiber density was lower in DM patients with refractory scalp pruritus compared with normal control patients in posterior parietal and occipital scalp areas, suggesting the possibility of a scalp neuropathy in the DM patients.[23] Additionally, it was just shown IL-31 levels correlate highly with pruritus and cutaneous disease activity in DM patients, and itch improvement correlated with significant reductions in IL-31 in DM lesional skin.[24] Whether specifically targeting IL-31 in refractory patients is an effective strategy for DM remains to be seen, but appears promising.

CUTANEOUS LUPUS ERYTHEMATOSUS

Cutaneous involvement of lupus erythematosus (LE) can occur as the sole manifestation of disease, but also represents the second most common organ involved in systemic LE (SLE).[25] Although most dermatologists are familiar with the subtypes of cutaneous LE (CLE), there is a consensus that it remains an ill-defined disease. Classification criteria that more objectively defines CLE and helps clinicians to distinguish CLE from other mimics is lacking, and this shortcoming is likely impeding both optimal clinical care and ability to adequately conduct clinical studies. Recently, there has been significant activity to address these inadequacies, first focusing on discoid LE. A Delphi consensus exercise performed by a group of CLE experts determined 12 clinical and histologic criteria for potential inclusion into discoid LE classification criteria.[26] Currently, studies to assess these 12 clinical and histologic criteria in discoid LE versus other mimicker diseases is underway. In the future, similar studies to develop criteria for other CLE subtypes may be performed.

There has also been significant progress in better understanding the pathogenesis of CLE. The type I IFN inflammatory environment in CLE is known to be driven by both plasmacytoid dendritic cells and keratinocytes.[27] Additionally, it is thought the accumulation of apoptotic cells is fundamental to both SLE and CLE pathogenesis.[28] Recent evidence suggests, in a background of lupus immunologic dysregulation, that UV irradiation can contribute to pathogenic accumulation of apoptotic cells in the skin.[29] This accumulation of apoptotic material, coupled with impaired ability to clear cellular debris, leads to secondary necrosis of apoptotic cells and the release of large quantities of endogenous nucleic acids (eNA).[30]

Strong evidence that eNA may play a pathogenic role in chronic CLE inflammation was also demonstrated.[29] eNA can strongly induce keratinocytes to release CXCL10 and IFN-regulated cytokines. CXCL10 expression then drives recruitment of $CXCR3^+$ cytotoxic immune cells to induce vacuolar interface dermatitis and further keratinocyte death. This process propagates the release of more eNA motifs to fuel and sustain chronic inflammation and development of chronic CLE lesions. eNAs from dying cells seem to induce keratinocyte production of proinflammatory cytokines, in particular, through activation of pathogen recognition receptor pathways via nucleic acids.[29] LL-37 (cathelicidin), which is expressed in CLE lesions, may act as a transfectant to introduce eNAs into keratinocytes and help to trigger this inflammatory cascade.

Another study suggests keratinocytes may be inherently primed by IFN-κ to produce abundant amounts of IL-6 in the setting of CLE.[31] Thus, a predisposition for brisk type I IFN inflammatory responses by lupus keratinocytes upon stimulation may exist owing to an autocrine loop involving IFN-κ. This may be a mechanism by which environmental factors such as UV exposure trigger robust inflammatory responses and release of eNA leading to CLE development.

Currently, antimalarials are considered first-line systemic treatment for CLE. There are 3 antimalarials commonly used to treat CLE: hydroxychloroquine (HCQ), chloroquine (CQ), and quinacrine. Quinacrine may be underused owing to its lack of availability. However, although quinacrine is currently not manufactured by any company, it can be compounded into capsules readily by most compounding pharmacies. Quinacrine has the advantage of not being associated with retinal toxicity, unlike HCQ and CQ. Studies have also suggested quinacrine may be a stronger antiinflammatory agent than HCQ or CQ, and recently it was shown to more effectively suppress both tumor necrosis factor-α and IFN-α in peripheral blood mononuclear cells from patients with DM and CLE.[32,33]

Importantly, multiple studies have been performed recently that can potentially be translated into safer and more effective use of antimalarials for CLE in everyday clinical practice. A major update concerns dosing and retinal toxicity screening for HCQ. Based on a cohort of 2361 patients who had been exposed to antimalarials, it was found HCQ doses of ≤5.0 mg/kg actual body weight were associated with significantly less retinal toxicity risk compared with higher doses.[34] This study triggered new recommendations from the American Academy of Ophthalmology to limit HCQ dosing to ≤5 mg/kg actual body weight.[35] This dosing is similar to previous recommendations (<6.5 mg/kg ideal body weight) for many patients, but seems to be most important for very thin patients who otherwise may have taken doses placing them at high retinal toxicity risk. These new recommendations are controversial for obese patients, however.

Additionally, the American Academy of Ophthalmology recommends, following a baseline examination for retinal toxicity within the first 12 months of treatment, that a repeat screening examination is not required until a patient has been taking HCQ for 5 years, assuming the patient has normal retinal toxicity risk.[35] This recommendation is based on research supporting cumulative HCQ dose is the most important risk factor for retinal toxicity, and most patients who have developed retinal toxicity have taken cumulative doses of 1000 g or more, which would occur if a patient takes 400 mg/d for 7 years. Although these guidelines are also not without controversy, it is important for clinicians who prescribe antimalarials to be knowledgeable about them.

Despite being well-recognized as first-line treatment, the first double-blind, randomized trial comparing HCQ with placebo in CLE was only recently reported.[36] The primary endpoint of decrease in Cutaneous Lupus Activity and Severity Index after 16 weeks was met, but did not significantly differ in the HCQ versus placebo groups. However, Physician Global Assessment, pain, and fatigue scores did significantly improve in the HCQ group compared with the placebo group at week 16, supporting the effectiveness of HCQ for CLE and its first-line treatment status.

Several studies concerning optimizing use of antimalarials for CLE are worth noting. In 1 study, researchers examined usefulness of switching antimalarials after patients either (1) failed to respond or (2) had an adverse reaction to a first antimalarial.[37] They found >50% of patients responded to a second antimalarial after failing the first, although the response seemed to decrease with time. Additionally, 69% of patients exposed to a second antimalarial agent after having an adverse reaction to the first tolerated it without incident. Furthermore, 80% of the patients who tolerated the second antimalarial responded positively to it. Additional studies suggest adding quinacrine to either HCQ or CQ can be a useful strategy for up to two-thirds of patients who fail either medication as monotherapy.[38,39] Adding quinacrine to either HCQ or CQ seems not only to be effective, but also safe. Thus, switching antimalarials and/or adding quinacrine before exposing patients with CLE to more toxic immunosuppressive medications seems to be an important treatment consideration.

There continues to be mounting evidence suggesting measurement of whole blood HCQ levels can be clinically important, because they are correlated with response in patients with CLE.[40] This finding raises the obvious question concerning whether clinicians should simply dose HCQ to reach adequate whole blood levels on an individual basis. Chasset and colleagues[41] recently explored this possibility. They increased daily HCQ dose (maximum 800 mg/d) in 32 patients with refractory CLE until HCQ blood concentrations were greater than 750 ng/mL. With this strategy, 26 patients (81%) reached the primary endpoint of significant improvement in Cutaneous Lupus Activity and Severity Index activity. However, the median daily HCQ dose required to achieve blood levels of greater than 750 ng/mL was 9.8 mg/kg actual body weight (range, 6.8–13.8 mg/kg actual body weight) and 9.2 mg/kg ideal body weight (range, 5.7–14.5 mg/kg ideal body weight), which is significantly higher than current or past recommended safe dosing. Although many patients were able to eventually decrease dosing to 400 mg/d, the authors note that this strategy may be preferable only in patients who have received a cumulative HCQ dose of less than 1000 g and that it is probably important to limit the time during which increased doses are used.

Despite these useful updates, a percentage of patients with CLE will not respond adequately to antimalarials. In this case, more traditional immunosuppressive medications should be considered. A recent study looking at effective treatments in patients with CLE who failed antimalarials found thalidomide to be particularly effective compared with other options.[42] Lenalidamide is a derivative of thalidomide that has also been shown to be effective for CLE.[43,44] Lenalidamide attractively lacks an association with peripheral neuropathy, which occurs in approximately 16% of CLE patients who take thalidomide for extended periods of time.[45]

There is an abundance of activity regarding a search for more effective CLE treatments. A novel thalidomide-like medication has recently been shown to more effectively decrease Aiolos, a protein implicated in promoting LE disease activity, levels than either thalidomide or lenalidamide.[46] Results of a phase IIa study suggest promising efficacy in patients with SLE, and a phase IIb study is underway in a larger SLE patient population.[47,48] Because skin activity improved in patients enrolled in the phase IIa study, specifically examining efficacy and safety of this medication for CLE should be considered.

Although a phase I study lacked impressive results, there was improvement in a number of endpoints, including Cutaneous Lupus Activity and Severity Index scores, in a phase IIb study evaluating treatment with the anti–IFN-α monoclonal antibody, sifalimumab, in patients with SLE.[49,50] However, more promising improvements in CLE were seen in a recent phase IIb clinical trial assessing efficacy of anifrolumab, an anti-type I IFN receptor monoclonal antibody, in patients with SLE.[51] In light of this finding, sifalimumab production has been discontinued and immediate future studies will focus on anifrolumab in LE.[22] Additional ongoing clinical trials for novel CLE treatments are listed in **Table 1**.

MORPHEA

There are numerous fibrosing skin diseases treated by dermatologists. Most are challenging to treat and may have devastating negative effects on patients' quality of life. Thus, there is a great need for a better understanding of pathogenesis and better treatments for this group of conditions. Given the limitations of this review, here we focus on updates concerning localized scleroderma, or morphea.

Numerous advancements in the clinical aspects of morphea have occurred in the past few years.

Table 1
Survey of current clinical trials focused on treatment of cutaneous lupus erythematosus

Study Title	Intervention	ClinicalTrials.Gov Identifier
Treatment of Cutaneous Lupus Erythematosus (CLE) With the 595 nm Flashlamp Pulsed Dye Laser	595 nm flashlamp pulsed dye laser	NCT00523588
Safety and Efficacy of Filgotinib and GS-9876 in Females With Moderately-to-Severely Active Cutaneous Lupus Erythematosus (CLE)	JAK 1 inhibitor	NCT03134222
To Evaluate the Preliminary Safety, Tolerability, Pharmacokinetics, Pharmacodynamics and Efficacy of CC-11050 in Subjects With Discoid Lupus Erythematosus and Subacute *Cutaneous Lupus* Erythematosus	Phosphodiesterase-4 inhibitor	NCT01300208
Low-dose UVA1 Radiation in Cutaneous Lupus Patients	UVA-1 phototherapy 20 J/cm^2 3 times per week	NCT01776190
IVIg Efficacy Study to Treat Lupus Erythematosus	2 g/kg/mo IVIg	NCT01841619
Study to Evaluate BIIB059 in Cutaneous Lupus Erythematosus (CLE) With or Without Systemic Lupus Erythematosus (SLE)	Monoclonal antibody targeting blood dendritic cell antigen 2 (BDCA2)	NCT02847598
Safety and Efficacy of KRP203 in Subacute Cutaneous Lupus Erythematosus	Sphingosine 1 phosphate receptor agonist	NCT01294774
Safety, Tolerability, Pharmacokinetics, Pharmacodynamics and Clinical Effect of GSK2646264 in Cutaneous Lupus Erythematosus Patients	Topical SYK inhibitor	NCT02927457
Open-label Study of Tofacitinib for Moderate to Severe Skin Involvement in Young Adults With Lupus	JAK1/2/3 inhibitor	NCT03288324
Safety and Efficacy of Topical R333 in Patients With Discoid Lupus Erythematosus (DLE) and Systemic Lupus Erythematosus (SLE) Lesions	Topical dermatologic JAK/SYK inhibitor	NCT01597050

Select Clinical Trials listed as Active or Completed on ClinicalTrials.Gov with search terms "cutaneous lupus" on June 27, 2018.
Abbreviations: IVIg, intravenous immunoglobulin; JAK, Janus kinase; SYK, spleen tyrosine kinase.

Generalized morphea is a relatively common morphea subtype and one of the most severe. However, the criteria for diagnosing generalized morphea differ in various classification schemes, most of which are not based on well-studied prospective cohorts.[52,53] This variability can impede clinical care and research, akin to CLE described earlier. Recently, Teske and colleagues[54] used computerized lesion mapping to objectively determine the cutaneous distribution of lesions in patients with generalized morphea. Their analysis suggests there are 3 groups of generalized morphea patients with distinct clinical and demographic features. They propose patients with generalized morphea be categorized as having either isomorphic or symmetric subtypes and that patients with multiple linear lesions be excluded from generalized morphea classification. This classification could allow for more homogenous populations to better study the genetics, pathogenesis, and treatment of this heterogenous disease.

Useful biomarkers and other clues predicting morphea clinical activity are also lacking. It has recently been demonstrated patients with morphea have increased myelin basic protein (MBP) serum levels and anti-MBP antibodies, and those with anti-MBP antibodies have increased levels of pain and histologic perineural inflammation in skin.[55] This finding suggests anti-MBP antibodies to be a potentially useful biomarker for severe morphea and a target for mechanistic studies, but additional research is needed. Another study systematically evaluated the histologic features in morphea lesional skin biopsies and their relationship with clinical features.[56] It was found bottom-heavy patterns of sclerosis and severe inflammation both were associated with patient perceived pain and tightness. This finding suggests value in describing detailed histologic features in morphea pathology reports and implies such patients with these histologic features may require more aggressive monitoring and treatment.

Other potential biomarkers were identified recently by evaluating cytokine levels in whole blood and morphea lesional skin and comparing these with healthy control subjects.[57] CXCL9 was found to be significantly elevated in morphea serum and levels correlated with disease activity severity. Double-staining immunohistochemistry revealed CXCL9 colocalized with CD68+ dermal macrophages, implying from a pathogenesis standpoint that skin may be the source of circulating cytokines. CXCL10, in contrast, may be a marker of overall sclerosis severity. Furthermore, morphea patient serum revealed evidence of Th1 IFN-γ imbalances, but absence of a transcriptional IFN signature in the peripheral blood. This finding differs from that seen in systemic sclerosis (SSc), suggesting skin fibrosis in these diseases may result from different processes.

These findings are particularly interesting because it has been noted some patients with SSc develop classic morphea lesions.[58] Although the percentage of patients with SSc who developed morphea lesions was low (12 of 370 [3.2%]), it is notable some developed morphea (especially generalized morphea) before SSc diagnosis. Also of note, Raynaud's phenomenon and nailfold capillary changes were universally present in these patients with SSc, suggesting clinical features can help to distinguish between these diseases. Another study examined anatomic distribution of pediatric-onset morphea lesions.[59] This study revealed morphea disproportionately affects the hands, feet, extensor extremities, posterior trunk, and upper face. Because these areas may be more prone to trauma, the findings support the theory that trauma is an etiologic factor in morphea pathogenesis.

Although classically thought to be a disease isolated to skin and occasionally involving the subcutis and/or fascia, a recent study explored the association between morphea and inflammatory arthritis.[60] The authors found 11 of 53 pediatric morphea patients (21%) had polyarthritis, and involved joints were unrelated to sites of morphea. This finding is in line with a previous study of 750 pediatric morphea patients in which 22% of patients had extracutaneous manifestations, with articular disease being the most common.[61] The joints most commonly affected were the proximal interphalangeal and metacarpophalangeal joints of the fingers (10 of 11 patients).[60] Antinuclear antibody positivity was significantly higher in patients with arthritis (8 of 10) compared with patients without arthritis (8 of 21).

Finally, there have been few studies evaluating how morphea affects health-related quality of life and these have yielded conflicting results. A more recent study in adults with morphea showed it significantly impaired health-related quality of life, most prominently in terms of emotional well-being and concerns the disease would progress to internal organs.[62] This finding has importance for providers who care for morphea patients, especially in terms of evaluation and education.

Treatment of morphea is not well-defined and a recent survey study suggests there is large variation in how pediatric dermatologists treat pediatric morphea.[63] In another survey, dermatologists generally reported preference for topical treatments, whereas rheumatologists reported preference for using systemic immunosuppressives.[64] In this latter survey, however, pediatric dermatologists were more closely aligned with pediatric rheumatologists in their use of systemic medications. Studies have also shown outcomes differ depending on timing of morphea onset. Although many patients with pediatric-onset morphea will experience disease activity into adulthood, patients with morphea onset in adulthood may have increased disease severity.[65]

Topical and systemic glucocorticoids with or without methotrexate represent the mainstay of treatment for morphea subtypes, but several recent reports suggest novel morphea treatments may be emerging. One of these is abatacept, a recombinant fusion protein composed of an Fc region of IgG1 fused to the extracellular domain of CTLA-4. There have been 2 reports published that describe a total of 5 patients with deep morphea who were treated successfully with abatacept.[66,67] In one of the reports describing 3 patients, the mean Modified Rodnan Skin Score improved dramatically from baseline by 37% at 6 months and 74% at 18 months.[66]

In 2 other reports, a total of 7 children between 6 and 13 years of age with morphea were treated with tocilizumab, an anti–IL-6 monoclonal antibody that has shown promise for treating SSc.[68] Tocilizumab treatment resulted in significantly improved Physician Global Assessment scores, but not changes in the Modified Localized Scleroderma Skin Activity Index in 1 report.[69] In the other report, 2 children with pansclerotic morphea were treated with tocilizumab and experienced significant decreases in Modified Localized Scleroderma Skin Activity Index scores.[70]

Finally, UVA-1 phototherapy has shown efficacy in treating morphea and other fibrosing skin diseases in numerous studies.[71,72] A more recent prospective study revealed 60% of patients with morphea (37 of 62 patients) were responders to UVA-1, although 46% of responders (17 of 37 patients) had disease recurrence after UVA-1.[73] Given the relative safety of phototherapy compared with most systemic medications, additional studies aimed at optimizing beneficial effects of UVA-1 in morphea are needed.

CUTANEOUS VASCULITIS

The skin represents one of the most frequent organs affected by vasculitis. In patients with cutaneous vasculitis, multiple organ systems can be involved or the vasculitic process may be isolated to skin (skin-limited vasculitis). The 2012 revised International Chapel Hill Consensus Conference Nomenclature of Vasculitidies (CHCC2012) reflected updates in the understanding of vasculitis relative to the previous conference in 1994.[74] However, CHCC2012 did not address skin-limited or skin-predominant forms of vasculitis. In light of this deficiency, an expert consensus group convened to propose an addendum to CHCC2012 that focused on cutaneous vasculitidies.[75] This addendum, which importantly included many dermatologists, helps to clarify CHCC2012 categories applicable to skin vasculitis and adds definitions of cutaneous vasculitis not included in the CHCC2012. This work, similar to what is described in other disease states in this review, can help to better define patients enrolled in clinical trials and other research studies to optimize chances of better understanding and treating this subset of vasculitis patients.

Of vasculidities predominantly affecting the skin, arguably the most updates have occurred in recent years for IgA-mediated cutaneous vasculitis, also often referred to as Henoch-Schonlein purpura (HSP). The initial ACR diagnostic criteria for IgA-mediated vasculitis did not include direct immunofluorescence (DIF) findings of IgA deposits in cutaneous vessels.[76] However, more recent classification criteria such as CHCC2012 and EULAR/PRINTO/PRES 2010 have included this diagnostic criterion.[74,77] This update is important for the dermatology community, because finding IgA deposits in cutaneous vessels has classically been a key test used to distinguish IgA-mediated vasculitis from other vasculitidies in the dermatology clinic. In fact, recent research by our dermatopathology group suggests IgA is the most useful immunoreactant to use for DIF studies in patients with suspected cutaneous vasculitis.[78]

Two studies found perivascular IgM deposits in lesional skin DIF specimens to be associated with renal involvement in adults with IgA-mediated vasculitis,[79,80] whereas Poterucha and colleagues[81] did not identify this association. Although DIF predictors of renal involvement in adult HSP patients would be useful, the discrepancy in significant findings within these studies implies no finding is yet ready to trust as a predictor in routine clinical practice. Additionally, a recent study suggests the presence of linear purpura (≥3 cm in length) is often found in children with HSP (8 of 31 patients), suggesting this finding may be an important clinical clue to this diagnosis[82] (Fig. 2). Although interesting, future studies are needed to determine if this or any clinical finding can reproducibly be useful for predicting diagnosis of IgA-mediated cutaneous vasculitis/HSP or end-organ involvement other than the skin.

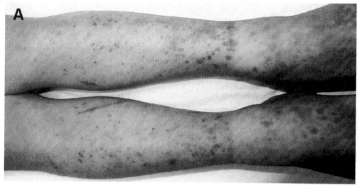
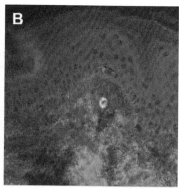

Fig. 2. (A) A 7-year-old boy presenting to clinic with purpura on the legs, including several areas on the upper legs and ankles of linear purpura (>3 cm in length). (B) A biopsy for hematoxylin and eosin staining displayed leukocytoclastic vasculitis (LCV; not shown), and direct immunofluorescence revealed granular deposition of IgA within superficial dermal blood vessel walls, compatible with IgA-mediated LCV/Henoch-Schonlein purpura (original magnification ×20).

There are few well-designed clinical studies that have investigated efficacy of treatments for cutaneous vasculitis. In fact, the only randomized, controlled study for cutaneous vasculitis was reported by Sais and colleagues[83] in 1995 and included 41 patients randomized to either oral colchicine 0.5 mg twice daily or topical emollients. In this study colchicine had no significant therapeutic effect compared with topical emollients. Thus, optimal treatment of cutaneous vasculitis remains unknown.

There are currently 2 ongoing studies that aim to improve not only our understanding of cutaneous vasculitis, but also identify more optimal treatment strategies. The Clinical Transcriptomics in Systemic Vasculitis (CUTIS) study will analyze molecular characteristics of vasculitic skin lesions across a variety of vasculitidies, including systemic forms.[84] Alternatively, the ARAMIS study (A Randomized Multicenter Study for Isolated Skin Vasculitis) will randomize patients with various skin-isolated, chronic vasculitic diseases to receive either colchicine, azathioprine, or dapsone to determine which of these agents, if any, is more effective for treatment.[85] Results of these studies will hopefully be available within the next few years and provide better clinical strategies for care of patients with skin-isolated vasculitis.

SUMMARY

This review highlights a wealth of activity aimed at better understanding and treating cutaneous disease associated with various connective tissue disorders. Thanks to the hard work and dedication of a growing group of dermatologist-researchers and other professionals, the future for patients who suffer from significant cutaneous manifestations of these diseases looks extremely bright.

ACKNOWLEDGMENTS

The author thanks Janine Sot for her expertise in preparing the figures for this article.

REFERENCES

1. Lundberg IE, Tjarnlund A, Bottai M, et al. 2017 European League Against Rheumatism/American College of Rheumatology classification criteria for adult and juvenile idiopathic inflammatory myopathies and their major subgroups. Arthritis Rheumatol 2017;69:2271–82.
2. Bohan A, Peter JB. Polymyositis and dermatomyositis (first of two parts). N Engl J Med 1975;292:344–7.
3. Bohan A, Peter JB. Polymyositis and dermatomyositis (second of two parts). N Engl J Med 1975;292:403–7.
4. Patel B, Khan N, Werth VP. Applicability of EULAR/ACR classification criteria for dermatomyositis to amyopathic disease. J Am Acad Dermatol 2018;79:77–83.e1.
5. Bailey EE, Fiorentino DF. Amyopathic dermatomyositis: definitions diagnosis and management. Curr Rheumatol Rep 2014;16:465.
6. Robinson ES, Feng R, Okawa J, et al. Improvement in the cutaneous disease activity of patients with dermatomyositis is associated with a better quality of life. Br J Dermatol 2015;172:169–74.
7. Huber AM, Kim S, Reed AM, et al. Childhood arthritis and rheumatology research alliance consensus clinical treatment plans for juvenile dermatomyositis with persistent skin rash. J Rheumatol 2017;44:110–6.
8. Sanner H, Sjaastad I, Flatø B. Disease activity and prognostic factors in juvenile dermatomyositis: a longterm follow-up study applying the Paediatric Rheumatology International Trials Organization criteria for inactive disease and the myositis disease

activity assessment tool. Rheumatology (Oxford) 2014;53:1578–85.

9. Seshadri R, Feldman BM, Ilowite N, et al. The role of aggressive corticosteroid therapy in patients with juvenile dermatomyositis: a propensity score analysis. Arthritis Rheum 2008;59:989–95.

10. Wolstencroft PW, Chung L, Li S, et al. Factors associated with clinical remission of skin disease in dermatomyositis. JAMA Dermatol 2018;154:44–51.

11. Hornung T, Janzen V, Heidgen FJ, et al. Remission of recalcitrant dermatomyositis treated with ruxolitinib. N Engl J Med 2014;371:2537–8.

12. Kurtzman DJ, Wright NA, Lin J, et al. Tofacitinib citrate for refractory cutaneous dermatomyositis: an alternative treatment. JAMA Dermatol 2016;152: 944–5.

13. Aggarwal R, Marder G, Koontz DC, et al. Efficacy and safety of adrenocorticotropic hormone gel in refractory dermatomyositis and polymyositis. Ann Rheum Dis 2018;77:720–7.

14. Efficacy and Safety of H.P. Acthar Gel for the Treatment of Refractory Cutaneous Manifestations of Dermatomyositis (Acthar Gel). Available at: https://clinicaltrials.gov/ct2/show/NCT02245841. Accessed June 27, 2018.

15. Motwani MP, Bennett F, Norris PC, et al. Potent anti-inflammatory and pro-resolving effects of anabasum in a human model of self-resolving acute inflammation. Clin Pharmacol Ther 2017. [Epub ahead of print].

16. Werth VP, Hejazi E, Pena SM, et al. A phase 2 study of safety and efficacy of anabasum (JBT-101), a cannabinoid receptor type 2 agonist, in refractory skin-predominant dermatomyositis [abstract]. Arthritis Rheumatol 2017;69(suppl 10).

17. Werth VP, Patel B, Concha JS, et al. SAT0512 Safety and efficacy of lenabasum in refractory skin-predominant dermatomyositis subjects treated in an open label extension of trial JBT101-DM-001. Ann Rheum Dis 2018;77(Suppl 2):1111–2.

18. Huard C, Gulla SV, Bennett DV, et al. Correlation of cutaneous disease activity with type 1 interferon gene signature and interferon B in dermatomyositis. Br J Dermatol 2017;176:1224–30.

19. Wong D, Kea B, Pesich R, et al. Interferon and biologic signatures in dermatomyositis skin: specificity and heterogeneity across diseases. PLoS One 2012;7:e29161.

20. Liao AP, Salajegheh M, Nazareno R, et al. Interferon beta is associated with type 1 interferon-inducible gene expression in dermatomyositis. Ann Rheum Dis 2011;70:831–6.

21. Higgs BW, Zhu W, Morehouse C, et al. A phase 1b clinical trial evaluating sifalimumab, an anti-IFN-α monoclonal antibody, shows target neutralisation of a type I IFN signature in blood of dermatomyositis and polymyositis patients. Ann Rheum Dis 2014; 73(1):256–62.

22. Adis Insight. Sifalimumab. Available at: https://adisinsight.springer.com/drugs/800024071.

23. Cirino P, Romiti R, McAdams B, et al. Scalp neuropathy in dermatomyositis patients with recalcitrant scalp pruritus. J Invest Dermatol 2018;138(5, Suppl):S74.

24. Kim HJ, Bonciani D, Zeidi M, et al. Itch in dermatomyositis: the role of increased skin interleukin-31. Br J Dermatol 2018. [Epub ahead of print].

25. Obermoser G, Sontheimer RD, Zelger B. Overview of common, rare and atypical manifestations of cutaneous lupus erythematosus and histopathological correlates. Lupus 2010;19(9):1050–70.

26. Elman SA, Joyce C, Nyberg F, et al. Development of classification criteria for discoid lupus erythematosus: results of a delphi exercise. J Am Acad Dermatol 2017;77:261–7.

27. Wenzel J, Tuting T. An IFN-associated cytotoxic cellular immune response against viral, self-, or tumor antigens is a common pathogenetic feature in "interface dermatitis". J Invest Dermatol 2008;128: 2392e402.

28. Kuhn A, Wenzel J, Bijl M. Lupus erythematosus revisited. Semin Immunopathol 2016;38:97–112.

29. Scholtissek B, Zahn S, Maier J, et al. Immunostimulatory endogenous nucleic acids drive the lesional inflammation in cutaneous lupus erythematosus. J Invest Dermatol 2017;137:1484–92.

30. Mahajan A, Herrmann M, Munoz LE. Clearance deficiency and cell death pathways: a model for the pathogenesis of SLE. Front Immunol 2016;7:35.

31. Stannard JN, Reed TJ, Myers E, et al. Lupus skin is primed for IL-6 inflammatory responses through a keratinocytes-mediated autocrine type I interferon loop. J Invest Dermatol 2017;137:115–22.

32. Wallace DJ. The use of quinacrine (Atrabine) in rheumatic diseases: a reexamination. Semin Arthritis Rheum 1989;18:282–97.

33. Alves P, Bashir MM, Wysocka M, et al. Quinacrine suppresses tumor necrosis factor-α and IFN-α in dermatomyositis and cutaneous lupus erythematosus. J Investig Dermatol Symp Proc 2017;18: S57–63.

34. Melles RB, Marmor MF. The risk of toxic retinopathy in patients on long-term hydroxychloroquine therapy. JAMA Ophthalmol 2014;132:1453–60.

35. Marmor MF, Kellner U, Lai TYY, et al. Recommendations on screening for chloroquine and hydroxychloroquine retinopathy (2016 revision). Ophthalmology 2016;123:1386–94.

36. Yokogawa N, Eto H, Tanikawa A, et al. Effects of hydroxychloroquine in patients with cutaneous lupus erythematosus: a multicenter, double-blind, randomized, parallel-group trial. Arthritis Rheumatol 2017; 69:791–9.

37. Chasset F, Arnaud L, Jachiet M, et al. Changing antimalarial agents after inefficacy or intolerance in

patients with cutaneous lupus erythematosus: a multicenter observational study. J Am Acad Dermatol 2018;78:107–14.

38. Chang AY, Piette EW, Foering KP, et al. Response to antimalarial agents in cutaneous lupus erythematosus: a prospective analysis. Arch Dermatol 2011; 147:1261–7.

39. Chasset F, Bouaziz JD, Costedoat-Chalumeau N, et al. Efficacy and comparison of antimalarials in cutaneous lupus erythematosus subtypes: a systematic review and meta-analysis. Br J Dermatol 2017;177:188–96.

40. Frances C, Cosnes A, Duhaut P, et al. Low blood concentration of hydroxychloroquine in patients with refractory cutaneous lupus erythematosus: a French multicenter prospective study. Arch Dermatol 2012;148:479–84.

41. Chasset F, Arnaud L, Costedoat-Chalumeau N, et al. The effect of increasing the dose of hydroxychloroquine (HCQ) in patients with refractory cutaneous lupus erythematosus (CLE): an open-label prospective pilot study. J Am Acad Dermatol 2016;74:693–9.

42. Fruchter R, Kurtzman DJB, Patel M, et al. Characteristics and alternative treatment outcomes of antimalarial-refractory cutaneous lupus erythematosus. JAMA Dermatol 2017;153:937–9.

43. Kindle SA, Wetter DA, Davis MDP, et al. Lenalidomide treatment of cutaneous lupus erythematosus: the Mayo Clinic experience. Int J Dermatol 2016; 55:e431–9.

44. Fennira F, Chasset F, Soubrier M, et al. Lenalidomide for refractory chronic and subacute cutaneous lupus erythematosus: 16 patients. J Am Acad Dermatol 2016;74:1248–51.

45. Chasset F, Tounsi T, Cesbron E, et al. Efficacy and tolerance profile of thalidomide in cutaneous lupus erythematosus: a systematic review and meta-analysis. J Am Acad Dermatol 2018;78:342–50.

46. Nakayama Y, Kosek J, Capone L, et al. Aiolos overexpression in systemic lupus erythematosus B cell subtypes and BAFF-induced memory B cell differentiation are reduced by CC-220 modulation of cereblon activity. J Immunol 2017;199:2388–407.

47. Werth VP, Furie R, Gaudy A, et al. CC-220 decreases B-cell subsets and plasmacytoid dendritic cells in systemic lupus erythematosus (SLE) patients and is associated with skin improvement: pharmacodynamic results from a phase IIa proof of concept study. (abstract) Arthritis Rheumatol 2017;69(suppl 10). Available at: https://acrabstracts.org/abstract/cc-220-decreases-b-cell-subsets-and-plasmacytoid-dendritic-cells-in-systemic-lupus-erythematosus-sle-patients-and-is-associated-with-skin-improvement-pharmacodynamic-results-from-a-phase-iia-proof/. Accessed June 29, 2018.

48. A Study to Evaluate the Efficacy and Safety of CC-220 in Subjects With Active Systemic Lupus Erythematosus. Available at: https://clinicaltrials.gov/ct2/show/NCT03161483.

49. Petri M, Wallace DJ, Spindler A, et al. Sifalimumab, a human anti-interferon-α monoclonal antibody, in systemic lupus erythematosus: a phase I randomized, controlled, dose-escalation study. Arthritis Rheum 2013;65:1011–21.

50. Khamashta M, Merrill JT, Werth VP, et al. Sifalimumab, an anti-interferon-α monoclonal antibody, in moderate to severe systemic lupus erythematosus: a randomised, double-blind, placebo-controlled study. Ann Rheum Dis 2016;75:1909–16.

51. Furie R, Khamashta M, Merrill JT, et al. CD1013 study investigators. anifrolumab, an anti-interferon-α receptor monoclonal antibody, in moderate-to-severe systemic lupus erythematosus. Arthritis Rheumatol 2017;69:376–86.

52. Peterson LS, Nelson AM, Su WP. Classification of morphea (localized scleroderma). Mayo Clin Proc 1995;70:1068–76.

53. Laxer RM, Zulian F. Localized scleroderma. Curr Opin Rheumatol 2006;18:606–13.

54. Teske N, Welser J, Jacobe H. Skin mapping for the classification of generalized morphea. J Am Acad Dermatol 2018;78:351–7.

55. Burger E, Paniagua R, Monson N, et al. Myelin basic protein antibodies as a biomarker in Morphea. J Invest Dermatol 2018;138(5 Suppl):S5.

56. Walker D, Susa JS, Currimbhoy S, et al. Histopathological changes in morphea and their clinical correlates: results from the Morphea in adults and children cohort V. J Am Acad Dermatol 2017;76: 1124–30.

57. O'Brien JC, Rainwater YB, Malviya N, et al. Transcriptional and cytokine profiles identify CXCL9 as a biomarker of disease activity in Morphea. J Invest Dermatol 2017;137:1663–70.

58. Chen JK, Chung L, Fiorentino DF. Characterization of patients with clinical overlap of morphea and systemic sclerosis: a case series. J Am Acad Dermatol 2016;74:1272–4.

59. Kiguradze T, Anderson K, Siddalb C, et al. Body site distribution of pediatric-onset morphea. J Invest Dermatol 2018;138(5 Suppl):S57.

60. Kashem SW, Correll CK, Vehe RK, et al. Inflammatory arthritis in pediatric patients with morphea. J Am Acad Dermatol 2018;79(1):47–51.e2.

61. Zulian F, Vallongo C, Woo P, et al. Localized scleroderma in childhood is not just a skin disease. Arthritis Rheum 2005;52(9):2873–81.

62. Klimas NK, Shedd AD, Bernstein IH, et al. Health-related quality of life in morphoea. Br J Dermatol 2015;172:1329–37.

63. Tollefson MM, Chiu YE, Brandling-Bennett HA, et al. Discordance of pediatric morphea treatment by pediatric dermatologists. Pediatr Dermatol 2018;35: 47–54.

64. Strickland N, Patel G, Strickland Am Jacobe H. Attitudes and trends in the treatment of morphea: a national survey. J Am Acad Dermatol 2015;72:727–8.

65. Condie D, Grabell D, Jacobe H. Comparison of outcomes in adults with pediatric-onset morphea and those with adult-onset Morphea. Arthritis Rheumatol 2014;66:3496–504.

66. Adeeb F, Anjum S, Hodnett P, et al. Early- and late-stage morphea subtypes with deep tissue involvement is treatable with Abatacept (Orencia). Semin Arthritis Rheum 2017;46:775–81.

67. Stausbøl-Grøn B, Olesen AB, Deleuran B, et al. Abatacept is a promising treatment for patients with disseminated morphea profunda: presentation of two cases. Acta Derm Venereol 2011;91:686–8.

68. Khanna D, Denton CP, Lin CJF, et al. Safety and efficacy of subcutaneous tocilizumab in systemic sclerosis: results from the open-label period of a phase II randomised controlled trial (faSScinate). Ann Rheum Dis 2018;77(2):212–20.

69. Lythgoe H, Baildam E, Beresford MW, et al. Tocilizumab as a potential therapeutic option for children with severe, refractory juvenile localized scleroderma. Rheumatology 2018;57:398–401.

70. Martini G, Campus S, Raffeiner B, et al. Tocilizumab in two children with pansclerotic morphoea: a hopeful therapy for refractory cases? Clin Exp Rheumatol 2017;35(Suppl. 106):S211–3.

71. Kreuter A, Hyun J, Stucker M, et al. A randomized controlled study of low-dose UVA1, medium-dose UVA1, and narrowband UVB phototherapy in the treatment of localized scleroderma. J Am Acad Dermatol 2006;54:440–7.

72. Andres C, Kollmar A, Mempel M, et al. Successful ultraviolet A1 phototherapy in the treatment of localized scleroderma: a retrospective and prospective study. Br J Dermatol 2010;162:445–7.

73. Vasquez R, Jabbar A, Khan F, et al. Recurrence of morphea after successful ultraviolet A1 phototherapy: a cohort study. J Am Acad Dermatol 2014;70:481–8.

74. Jennette JC, Falk RJ, Bacon PA, et al. 2012 revised International Chapel Hill Consensus Conference Nomenclature of Vasculitides. Arthritis Rheum 2013;65(1):1–11.

75. Sunderkötter CH, Zelger B, Chen KR, et al. Nomenclature of cutaneous vasculitis: dermatologic addendum to the 2012 Revised international chapel hill consensus conference nomenclature of vasculitides. Arthritis Rheumatol 2018;70:171–84.

76. Mills JA, Michel BA, Bloch DA, et al. The American College of Rheumatology 1990 criteria for the classification of vasculitis. Arthritis Rheum 1990;33:1114–21.

77. Ozen S, Pistorio A, Iusan SM, et al. EULAR/PRINTO/PRES criteria for Henoch–Schönlein purpura, childhood polyarteritis nodosa, childhood Wegener granulomatosis and childhood Takayasu arteritis: Ankara 2008. Part II: final classification criteria. Ann Rheum Dis 2010;69:798–806.

78. Feasel P, Billings SD, Bergfeld WF, et al. Direct immunofluorescence testing in vasculitis—A single institution experience with Henoch-Schönlein purpura. J Cutan Pathol 2018;45:16–22.

79. Poterucha TJ, Wetter DA, Gibson LE, et al. Correlates of systemic disease in adult Henoch-Schönlein purpura: a retrospective study of direct immunofluorescence and skin lesion distribution in 87 patients at Mayo Clinic. J Am Acad Dermatol 2012;67:612–6.

80. Takeuchi S, Soma Y, Kawakami T. IgM in lesional skin of adults with Henoch-Schönlein purpura is an indication of renal involvement. J Am Acad Dermatol 2010;63:1026–9.

81. Belli AA, Dervis E. The correlation between cutaneous IgM deposition and renal involvement in adult patients with Henoch-Schönlein purpura. Eur J Dermatol 2014;24:81–4.

82. Milani GP, Lava SAG, Ramelli V, et al. Prevalence and characteristics of nonblanching, palpable skin lesions with a linear pattern in children with Henoch-Schönlein syndrome. JAMA Dermatol 2017;153(11):1170–3.

83. Sais G, Vidaller A, Jucglà A, et al. Colchicine in the treatment of cutaneous leukocytoclastic vasculitis. Results of a prospective, randomized controlled trial. Arch Dermatol 1995;131(12):1399–402.

84. Clinical Transcriptomics in Systemic Vasculitis (CUTIS). Available at: https://clinicaltrials.gov/ct2/show/NCT03004326.

85. A Randomized Multicenter Study for Isolated Skin Vasculitis (ARAMIS). Available at: https://clinicaltrials.gov/ct2/show/NCT02939573.

Advances in Inflammatory Granulomatous Skin Diseases

Sotonye Imadojemu, MD, MBE, Misha Rosenbach, MD*

KEYWORDS

- Sarcoidosis - Necrobiosis lipoidica - Granuloma annulare - Reactive granulomatous dermatitis
- Biologics - Immunotherapy - Checkpoint inhibitors

KEY POINTS

- The etiopathogenesis of the inflammatory granulomatous disorders is not well understood.
- The T helper 1 (Th1) response mediated by interferon-gamma, tumor necrosis factor-alpha, and interleukin (IL) 1, 2, 6 and the T helper 17 response mediated by IL-17 play important roles in the development and maintenance of these diseases.
- Inflammatory granulomatous dermatitides are often associated with systemic diseases and have extracutaneous manifestations. Therefore, patients with these disorders require thorough evaluation to identify associated systemic findings.
- Anticancer therapies, such as immune-checkpoint inhibitors, have been associated with inflammatory granulomatous disease, which is enriching our understanding of the etiopathogenesis of and possible treatment avenues for inflammatory granulomatous dermatitides.

INTRODUCTION

The granulomatous dermatitides are a heterogenous group of conditions whose etiopathogenesis is poorly understood. Granulomas are organized collections of histiocytes. Histiocytes are divided into 2 groups: dendritic cells and mature macrophages. The primary function of dendritic cells is antigen presentation. Macrophages interact intimately with complement to recognize antigen and phagocytize antigen. Mature macrophages also secrete cytokines and chemokines, such as tumor necrosis factor (TNF) or interleukin-1 (IL-1). These cytokines influence both innate and adaptive immune responses, typically increasing inflammation in a nonspecific fashion, which may lead to fibrosis. Macrophages are in turn activated by cytokines, such as interferon-gamma (IFN-gamma) and TNF-alpha, leading to a positive feedback loop often leading to chronic inflammation. In this way, histiocytes interact with lymphocytes to create granulomas.

Granulomatous inflammation often arises in reaction to various triggers, such as foreign bodies, infections, metabolic disorders, environmental antigens, and malignancy. Granulomatous disorders are divided into those produced by known infectious causes and the inflammatory disorders, those without a known infectious cause. Infectious granulomatous diseases are outside the scope of this article. The inflammatory granulomatous diseases can be associated with an underlying systemic disease and sometimes represent a dysregulated immune system. In this article, the authors review 4 common inflammatory cutaneous

Disclosure statement: S. Imadojemu has nothing to disclose. M. Rosenbach has the following commercial or financial conflicts of interest and any funding sources to disclose: consultant, Processa Pharmaceuticals; past advisory board, Merck. Dr M. Rosenbach has received a Dermatology Foundation Medical Dermatology Career Development Award (for sarcoidosis/granulomatous diseases).
Dermatology Administration, Perelman Center for Advanced Medicine, University of Pennsylvania, 3400 Civic Center Boulevard, 7th Floor, South Tower, Philadelphia, PA 19104, USA
* Corresponding author.
E-mail address: Misha.rosenbach@uphs.upenn.edu

Dermatol Clin 37 (2019) 49–64
https://doi.org/10.1016/j.det.2018.08.001
0733-8635/19/© 2018 Elsevier Inc. All rights reserved.

granulomatous disorders (cutaneous sarcoidosis, necrobiosis lipoidica [NL], granuloma annulare, and reactive granulomatous dermatitis) and explore recent updates in the etiopathogenesis and management of these diseases.

REVIEW OF CUTANEOUS SARCOIDOSIS
Epidemiology

Sarcoidosis is a multiorgan disease that predominantly affects the lungs as well as the heart, eyes, upper airway, endocrine systems, and central nervous system. However, the skin is the second most frequently involved organ. Large and generalizable epidemiologic studies performed in the United States are needed to accurately comment on the incidence and prevalence of cutaneous sarcoidosis. An epidemiologic study performed in a predominantly Caucasian population in Minnesota from 1976 to 2013 found an annual age- and sex-adjusted incidence of sarcoidosis-specific skin lesions to be 1.9 per 100,000 population.[1] This finding is likely an underestimation of the overall true frequency of cutaneous sarcoidosis given the relative lack of racial diversity in this sample. The clinical presentation of cutaneous sarcoidosis may vary by ethnic background. African Americans have the highest rates of sarcoidosis in the United States and seem more likely to have chronic cutaneous sarcoidosis as compared with Caucasians.[2]

Etiopathogenesis

Sarcoidosis is a granulomatous disease characterized by dysregulation of the cell-mediated portion of the immune system.[3] It has been hypothesized that exposure to an antigen (environmental, infectious, or autoimmune) coupled with a genetic predisposition leads to activation of macrophages and T cells, with subsequent granuloma formation.[4] Tissue macrophages and T lymphocytes form granulomas with a fibrous capsule to surround pathogens to defend against a foreign antigen that cannot be easily cleared but for which cell-mediated immunity is intact. There are opposing paradigms for the pathogenesis for the granulomas of sarcoidosis as a hypoactive or hyperactive immune response to the yet unknown antigen. It may be that several triggers, such as mycobacteria, *Propionibacterium acnes*, a misfolded self-antigen, or organic or inorganic molecules from the environment, precipitate disease.[5–11] The increased incidence of involvement of organs that interact with the outside world, such as the skin, lungs, and eyes, supports a possible environmental trigger. Genetic susceptibility likely also plays a role. The immune profile of sarcoidosis is predominantly a T helper 1 (Th1) immune response with contributions of the innate and T

helper 17 arms of the immune system. Important cytokines in the pathophysiology of sarcoidosis include IL-1, IL-2, IL-6, IL-12, IL-17, IL-18; IFN-gamma; and TNF-alpha, with TNF-alpha and IFN-gamma consistently shown to play key roles.[12,13] These same cytokines have been implicated in many inflammatory granulomatous diseases.

Clinical and Histologic Presentation

Skin findings of systemic sarcoidosis develop before or at the time of diagnosis in 80% of patients.[14] There are specific and nonspecific findings of cutaneous sarcoidosis, based on the presence or absence of characteristic sarcoidal granulomas on biopsy. There are numerous clinical presentations of sarcoidosis-specific cutaneous disease, some common and some uncommon (**Fig. 1, Table 1**). The most common nonspecific cutaneous finding associated with sarcoidosis is erythema nodosum (EN). EN is a reactive inflammatory panniculitis and has been associated with a favorable prognosis in patients of Scandinavian European descent, often presenting as part of Löfgren syndrome.[15]

Histopathology of cutaneous sarcoidosis classically reveals superficial, deep dermal, and, occasionally, subcutaneous epithelioid granulomas, organized into tubercles, without a prominent surrounding lymphoplasmacytic infiltrate. Central necrosis or caseation is typically absent. Giant cells are typically present and may contain asteroid bodies or Schaumann bodies. Of note, up to 20% of biopsies of cutaneous sarcoidosis contain polarizable material.[16] Therefore, the presence of a foreign body does not exclude the diagnosis of sarcoidosis.

Evaluation and Management

Because sarcoidosis is a multiorgan systemic disease, the evaluation of patients with systemic sarcoidosis necessitates investigation for other

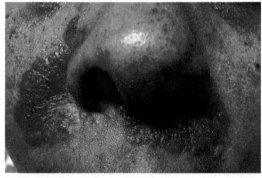

Fig. 1. Cutaneous sarcoidosis. Red-brown plaques on the cheeks and upper cutaneous lip.

Table 1
Common and uncommon specific cutaneous sarcoidosis findings

Common	Papules and papulonodules	• Most common morphology of the specific cutaneous manifestations of sarcoidosis • Description: numerous, firm, typically nonscaly papules usually smaller than 1 cm in size, rarely verrucous • Color: flesh colored, yellow-brown, red-brown, purple-brown, or hypopigmented • Location: typically on the face, often on the eyelids or alar rim, but also on the trunk and extremities
	Plaques	• Description: oval or annular, often well demarcated, typically firm to the touch and can sometimes have scale • Color: red-brown to flesh-colored to purple-brown and sometimes yellow-brown • Location: trunk, buttocks, shoulders, and arms
	Lupus pernio	• Can be disfiguring; tends to affect African Americans and women disproportionately; associated with a prolonged, chronic, and re-fractory course, often requiring aggressive systemic therapy • Description: smooth shiny plaques, which may develop scale • Color: brown to violaceous or pink-red • Location: central face, specifically the nose, cheeks, lips, forehead, also ears
	Subcutaneous nodules	• Description: firm, mobile, round to oval nodules • Color: erythematous, flesh-colored, violaceous, or brown. • Location: trunk and extremities, mainly upper extremities.
Uncommon	Ichthyosiform	• Fish scales, with adherent, polygonal, brown, or white-gray scale • Often located on the lower extremities
	Atrophic and ulcerative	• Depressed plaques, often ulcerate
	Mucosal	• Buccal mucosa, gingiva, hard palate, tongue, posterior pharynx, and salivary glands • Papules, plaques, nodules and localized edema; papules or infiltrative thickening
	Erythroderma	• Indurated, yellow-brown, red-brown or purple-brown scaly plaques coalesce to involve large areas of skin, often with fine superficial scale or mild exfoliative dermatitis
	Alopecic	• Scarring or nonscarring alopecia of the scalp
	Nail sarcoidosis	• Thinning, brittle nails, thickened nails, pitting, ridging, trachyo-nychia, hyperpigmentation, clubbing or pseudoclubbing, or destruction of the nail plate and scarring (pterygium)

organ involvement, including but not limited to pulmonary, cardiac, ophthalmologic, and endocrine disease (**Box 1**). Consultants, such as pulmonology, ophthalmology, otorhinolaryngology, cardiology, or rheumatology, may be necessary to manage the extracutaneous manifestations. A therapeutic regimen should be constructed to address the most severely affected organ and ideally should be crafted in a way that can help all affected organs. Control of cutaneous disease does not always correlate with control of extracutaneous disease. There are no Food and Drug Administration–approved therapies for cutaneous sarcoidosis. Treatment recommendations are based on small case series, retrospective studies, and expert opinion (**Table 2**). Cutaneous

sarcoidosis response to treatment is typically seen after 2 to 3 months of therapy and rarely sooner.

WHAT IS NEW IN CUTANEOUS SARCOIDOSIS
Sarcoidosis and Drug-Induced Sarcoidosis-like Reactions Due to Immune-Checkpoint Inhibitors

Immune-checkpoint inhibition with agents, such as ipilimumab, nivolumab, and pembrolizumab, are used to restore the antitumor T-cell response that is diminished by tumor-mediated mechanisms to evade the host immune response. These agents can lead to a durable antitumor immune response; however, they frequently cause

Box 1
Recommended evaluation and laboratory/imaging testing for patients with cutaneous sarcoidosis

History (including birth history, travel history, and occupational exposures)

Physical examination

Review of systems

Medication history

Laboratory and imaging tests:

- Chest radiograph
- Pulmonary function tests with diffusion capacity
- Ophthalmologic evaluation
- Complete blood count
- Comprehensive serum chemistries
- Electrocardiogram and transthoracic echocardiogram (or other dedicated testing, such as cardiac MRI, PET, or 24-hour Holter or event monitor depending on electrocardiogram and symptoms)
- Tuberculin skin test or IFN-gamma release assay
- Vitamin D25 and vitamin D1,25
- Thyroid-stimulating hormone

History, review of systems, and physical examination–driven laboratory and imaging studies

Table 2
Treatments for cutaneous sarcoidosis

Topical and local therapy	First-line agents: • Topical steroids • Intralesional corticosteroids • Topical calcineurin inhibitors Second-line agents: • Topical retinoids • Phototherapy and photodynamic therapy • Laser therapy with caution • Surgical excision with caution
Immunomodulatory systemic therapy	• Oral tetracycline antibiotics • Antimalarials • Phosphodiesterase inhibitors • Isotretinoin
Immunosuppressive systemic therapy	First-line agents: • Corticosteroids • Methotrexate • Antitumor necrosis factor agents (particularly infliximab, adalimumab) Second-line agents: • Repository corticotropin injection • Thalidomide and its derivatives • Mycophenolate mofetil • Azathioprine

immune-related adverse events (irAEs). These adverse events often include cutaneous eruptions, colitis, pneumonitis, and nephritis. There are many reports in the literature of patients with malignancy developing sarcoidosis and sarcoidosis-like drug reactions after anticancer therapy that can affect the skin, lungs, eyes, lymph nodes, and other organs.[17–22]

Idiopathic sarcoidosis is known to be associated with malignancy; the malignancy can present before, during, or long after the diagnosis of sarcoidosis. As discussed earlier, sarcoidosis may represent dysregulation of the immune system, possibly triggered by exposure to various antigens. In some instances, this dysregulation of the immune system may be triggered by, or develop as a response to, malignancy. Alternatively, it could be that chronic inflammation predisposes one to malignancy, specifically lymphoma.[23] Data on this topic have been inconsistent but largely favor an increased risk of malignancy in

those with sarcoidosis. However, it is important to note that this relationship has primarily been studied in European and Caucasian populations.[24–28]

Throughout the literature, there are many descriptive terms for the coincidence of sarcoidosis and malignancy. *Paraneoplastic sarcoidosis* is a term that has been used for the development of sarcoidal granulomas in 2 or more organs that emerges around the time of cancer presentation, follows the clinical course of the cancer, is refractory to conventional treatment, and responds to treatment of the cancer.[29] The co-occurence of sarcoidosis and neoplasia is quite rare, and the term *paraneoplastic sarcoidosis* is controversial; the primary association has been with lymphomas and lymphoproliferative disorders, rather than a broader association with malignancy.

In contrast, idiopathic sarcoidosis has been reported to be exacerbated by immune-checkpoint therapy. Cotliar and colleagues[20] report a case of a patient with a 12-year history of quiescent, asymptomatic sarcoidosis who developed refractory, stage IV Hodgkin lymphoma. She was treated with an immune-checkpoint inhibitor (ICI) and experienced an exacerbation of her underlying sarcoidosis with skin and pulmonary involvement. Furthermore, drug-induced sarcoidosis-like reactions (DISRs) have been reported after chemotherapy (cisplatin), targeted therapy (BRAF/MEK-inhibitors), or immunotherapy (IFN, IL-2, checkpoint inhibitors) for numerous malignancies in patients without a history of sarcoidosis.[17,19,21,22,30] It is these DISRs that the authors focus on, specifically ICI-associated reactions. Importantly, the authors argue that the term *sarcoidosis*, as a multiorgan disease, should be limited to those who have compatible clinical and radiologic findings supported by histologic evidence in one or more organs of noncaseating epithelioid-cell granulomas in the absence of microorganisms.[8] Notably, whether it is important to distinguish between sarcoidosis and sarcoidosis-like chemotherapy– or immunotherapy-associated (drug) reactions remains unclear.

Sarcoidosis-like lesions associated with ICIs may be clinically and radiographically concerning for disease recurrence or infection, which could significantly impact patient treatment.[18] Distinguishing between lymphoma progression and new sarcoidosis, and vice versa, is challenging. In those with preceding lymphoma, new sarcoidosis can be favored if lung disease, bilateral hilar lymphadenopathy (frequently asymptomatic), elevated angiotensin-converting enzyme level, and skin involvement are present.[31,32] In those with preceding sarcoidosis, new lymphoma can be favored if new lymph node disease, bone marrow, and splenic involvement are discovered.[31] Histologic confirmation is often necessary; excisional biopsy of the lymph node should be performed first. If not diagnostic, this test should be followed by bone marrow biopsy, endobronchial ultrasound-guided transbronchial needle aspiration, and then mediastinoscopy. Splenectomy and laparotomy should be considered last.[31]

Two large reviews of the literature on DISRs with ICIs have been performed and have similar findings.[18,22] Lung, hilar, and mediastinal nodes and skin were the most frequently involved organs in the ICI-associated sarcoidosis-like reactions with the average duration of therapy before the development of lesions of about 4.5 to 6.0 months (range: 0.75–20.0 months).[18,22]

Treatment of the sarcoidosis-like lesions included withholding therapy or administration of systemic steroids, and resolution or improvement occurred in 96% of patients irrespective of how the toxicity was treated.[18] Patients with an asymptomatic DISR with response to ICI therapy may benefit from continued treatment.[33] Those with mild to moderate DISR severity or those whose DISR is readily treatment responsive may also benefit from continued therapy with ICIs with close monitoring.

Additionally, the development of sarcoidosis-like lesions after ICI therapy seem to be another irAE that is associated with a favorable therapeutic response, although more data and longitudinal studies are necessary to verify this early observation.[18,22] Notably, there is a theoretical concern that treatment of irAEs with systemic steroids may offset some of the benefit of ICI therapy complicated by irAE. The use of targeted immunosuppressive agents or immunomodulatory agents, when possible, may lead to better outcomes. More research is needed on this topic.

New Insights in the Etiopathogenesis of Sarcoidosis

Finally, the multiple case reports and case series of the exacerbation of previously quiescent sarcoidosis and the development of sarcoidosis-like drug reactions have sparked interest in the role of programmed cell-death receptor (PD-1) and ligand (PD-L1) in the pathogenesis of idiopathic sarcoidosis. There is evidence to suggest that patients who develop idiopathic sarcoidosis, unrelated to ICI, may have a hypoactive immune response with decreased T-cell proliferation and PD-1 upregulation.[18,34] In a study of PD-L1 and PD-L2 expression in various benign and malignant histiocytic disorders, 7 of 7 cases (100%) of sarcoidosis lesions exhibited positivity for PD-L1 and PD-L2.[35] The research group headed by Drake found that patients with sarcoidosis have increased PD-1 expression on peripheral CD4+ T cells and increased expression of PD-L1 on sarcoidal granulomas.[36] Altogether, this suggests that the PD-1 receptor may play an important role in the pathogenesis of idiopathic sarcoidosis and that blockade of the PD-1 pathway may be a therapeutic target.[36] Notably, this is in contrast with the paradigm of a hyperactive immune response leading to ICI-associated sarcoidosis-like reactions discussed earlier. These findings suggest a different pathogenesis for idiopathic and ICI-associated sarcoidosis. This area of research continues to unfold.

REVIEW OF NECROBIOSIS LIPOIDICA
Epidemiology

NL is a chronic inflammatory granulomatous disease of the skin of unknown cause, seen most commonly, but not exclusively, in those with diabetes mellitus. It has been found that between 11% and 65% of patients with NL have diabetes mellitus or will go on to develop it.[37–40] However, among those with diabetes, those carrying a diagnosis of NL comprise only 0.3% to 1.2%.[37,41,42] NL occurs more frequently in women, with a female to male ratio of 3:1.[37,39,43] The average age of onset in those with diabetes-associated NL and non–diabetes-associated NL was 25 years and 46 years, respectively.[37] In addition to the association with diabetes, those with NL have an increased risk of thyroid disease (15.0%) as compared with the general population (5.5%).[39]

Etiopathogenesis

With regard to etiopathogenesis of NL, the strong association with diabetes mellitus has led to theories about the role of glycoprotein-mediated microangiopathy leading to tissue hypoxia, though there is some conflicting evidence about this relationship.[44–46] Another theory for the pathogenesis of NL is that the disease is due to abnormalities of collagen, as studies have found a decreased concentration and abnormal structure of collagen, possibly due to abnormal glucose metabolism in fibroblasts.[47,48] It is not known whether NL is a marker of the severity of diabetes mellitus or whether improved glycemic control leads to improvement in NL. It has been suggested that the presence of NL should prompt evaluation for other signs of end-organ damage, such as retinopathy, nephropathy, and neuropathy. These questions require further study.

Clinical and Histologic Presentation

The diagnosis of NL is made from a combination of clinical and histopathologic findings, as there is a robust clinical differential diagnosis for the disease. Clinical findings of NL include papules or plaques in the early stages of disease to atrophic patches or thin plaques. The color can be pink, brown, yellow-brown, red-brown, or yellow-orange depending on background skin color. NL often occurs on the pretibial leg but can occur on the scalp, face, trunk, and extremities. The atrophic patches and plaques are prone to ulcerations, often after minor trauma (**Fig. 2**). Histopathology of NL reveals palisaded and interstitial granulomas composed of histiocytes and multinucleated giant cells arranged in horizontal layers involving the

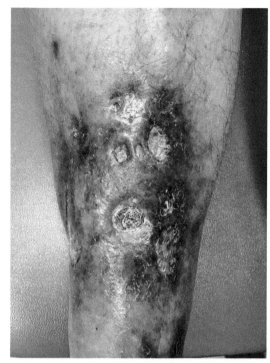

Fig. 2. NL complicated by minocycline hyperpigmentation. Atrophic and ulcerated gray-brown plaque on the anterior leg.

dermis and subcutis. There will be necrobiotic collagen in between the layers of granulomatous inflammation and often plasma cells at the dermal-subcutaneous junction and rarely lymphocytic aggregates in the deep dermis and subcutis. Skin biopsy should be obtained from the edge of the lesion and include subcutaneous fat to increase the chance of capturing diagnostic findings. The differential diagnosis includes granuloma annulare, cutaneous sarcoidosis (specifically the atrophic or ulcerative variants), and necrobiotic xanthogranuloma.

Evaluation and Management

Given the disease associations discussed earlier, patients with NL should be screened for diabetes and thyroid disease. There is a lack of high-quality data to support treatment recommendations for NL. There is no cure for the disease, though treatment may aid in halting progression as well as preventing and healing ulceration. The approach to treatment involves avoidance of trauma given the increased risk of ulceration in NL and minimizing inflammation with high-potency topical corticosteroids or intralesional corticosteroids. Corticosteroids should be applied or injected into the active, inflamed border that typically characterizes active NL and not to the atrophic areas. The primary side effect of topical and intralesional corticosteroids are atrophy, ulceration, and hypopigmentation.[49] Because atrophy and ulceration are manifestations of NL, close follow-up is necessary to prevent the development of corticosteroid-induced atrophy.

Other treatment options include, but are not limited to, topical tacrolimus, topical psoralen and ultraviolet A (PUVA) photochemotherapy, antimalarials, photodynamic therapy, pentoxifylline, TNF-alpha inhibitors, and fractional carbon dioxide laser therapy. Treatment of ulcerated NL involves the addition of basic wound care measures, optimization of nutrition, and control of lower extremity edema. Ulcerated necrobiosis therapy is challenging and often requires combination therapy.[50]

WHAT IS NEW IN NECROBIOSIS LIPOIDICA
Compilation of the Limited Data on Anti–Tumor Necrosis Factor-Alpha Agents for Necrobiosis Lipoidica

A recent review of reported cases of NL treated with anti–TNF-alpha agents included a total of 14 cases.[51] As discussed previously, anti–TNF-alpha agents can be helpful in granulomatous dermatitides given the role of TNF in granuloma formation and maintenance. Of the 14 reported cases, 5 were treated with systemic infliximab, 3 were treated with intralesional infliximab, 4 were treated with etanercept, and 2 with adalimumab. Eleven of the 14 cases resulted in marked improvement or complete remission of disease. The intervention with the least efficacy in this pooled sample of case reports/series were the 3 cases treated with intralesional infliximab. Intralesional infliximab resulted in reduction in erythema, reduction of pain, and healing of ulcers but persistence of plaques. Reported side effects were miliary tuberculosis, upper respiratory tract infections, and temporary fatigue.

Janus Kinase Pathway Inhibition for Necrobiosis Lipoidica

Abnormal activation of the Janus kinase/signal transducers and activators of transcription (JAK/STAT) pathway has been shown to be critical for the development of autoimmunity, hematologic malignancies, and aberrant hematopoietic stem cell development.[52] In dermatology, inhibition of the JAK/STAT pathway has been demonstrated to be useful in the treatment of cutaneous inflammatory diseases, such as psoriasis, atopic dermatitis, alopecia areata, and vitiligo.[53] Cytokines important for granuloma formation, such as IL-6,

IFN-gamma, and TNF-alpha, are known to be involved in the JAK/STAT pathway.[54–56] One recent report demonstrated dramatic improvement of treatment-refractory NL with the JAK-inhibitor ruxolitinib in a patient with polycythemia vera.[57] This finding suggests JAK-inhibitor therapy may prove beneficial in the treatment of NL and other inflammatory granulomatous diseases.

There is a paucity of high-quality data on the pathogenesis and effective treatment of NL, and more research is urgently needed.

REVIEW OF GRANULOMA ANNULARE
Epidemiology

Granuloma annulare (GA) is a noninfectious cutaneous granulomatous disease with many morphologies. There have been no population-based studies from which to obtain data on the incidence and prevalence of GA. It is a relatively uncommon disorder, as one review article reports that approximately 0.1% to 0.4% of new patients presenting to dermatologists were diagnosed with GA.[58] The female to male ratio is about 1 to 2:1.[59] There may be a bimodal distribution in age of patients presenting with GA. A Korean study described 44% of patients with GA present in the first decade of life and 44% present in the fifth decade of life.[60] GA is associated with various systemic diseases, including diabetes mellitus, thyroid dysfunction, dyslipidemia, chronic infections, and malignancy.[61]

Etiopathogenesis

The exact cause of the condition is unknown; but it has been hypothesized that GA is a reactive, cell-mediated, hypersensitivity to an unknown antigen. GA has been reported to occasionally emerge after exposure to possible triggers, including cutaneous trauma,[62] drugs,[63] vaccination,[64,65] and ultraviolet light exposure.[66] The cytokine profile is notable for increased expression of IFN-gamma, TNF-alpha, and matrix metalloproteinases, which degrade collagen. This milieu leads to activation of macrophages, IL-12–mediated differentiation of naïve T cells to the Th1 subtype, and IL-2–mediated recruitment of more T cells.[67,68]

Clinical and Histologic Presentation

Numerous clinical variants of GA have been described, including localized, generalized, subcutaneous, and numerous atypical presentations (**Fig. 3**). Localized GA is the classic presentation, comprising about 75% of reported cases of GA.[59] It is characterized by indurated papules, at times coalescing into plaques, often annular in

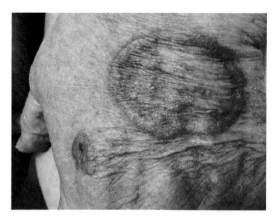

Fig. 3. Granuloma annulare. Pink-brown firm annular plaques on the dorsal hand.

configuration. Color is dark brown to purple skin in darker/deeper skin tones and skin colored to red-brown in fair to tan skin tones. Localized GA is often located on the hands and feet. Generalized GA is characterized by more widespread involvement, often of the trunk and extremities. The subcutaneous variant occurs nearly exclusively in children, typically on the lower extremities. Atypical presentations include the perforating, patch, palmoplantar, Blaschko linear, pustular, visceral, and annular elastolytic giant cell granuloma variants. On histology, there is mucin and palisading granulomatous inflammation surrounding degenerating collagen or interstitial granulomatous inflammation.

Evaluation and Management

Given the many systemic associations, further laboratory and imaging studies may be required (**Box 2**). GA is typically asymptomatic. Treatment is often indicated for cosmetic reasons (**Table 3**).

WHAT IS NEW IN GRANULOMA ANNULARE
Immunotherapy and Granuloma Annulare

Cancer immunology research developments have led to the widespread use of immunotherapy to treat solid and hematologic malignancies. Granulomatous dermatitis has been reported as a reaction to ICIs, such as PD-1 receptor and ligand inhibitors and cytotoxic T-lymphocyte antigen-4 inhibitors. As discussed earlier, PD-1 inhibitors block tumor-induced immunosuppression that cancers use to evade the immune system. The checkpoint inhibitors activate cytotoxic T cells to attack the tumor cell; however, these activated T cells may lead to immune dysregulation, autoimmunity, and subsequent organ dysfunction. Lichenoid and

---

> **Box 2**
> **Recommended evaluation and laboratory/imaging testing for patients with granuloma annulare**
>
> History and physical examination
>
> Review of systems
>
> Medication history
>
> Laboratory tests
> - Complete blood count with differential
> - Hemoglobin A1c
> - Thyroid-stimulating hormone
> - HIV antigen and antibody testing
> - Hepatitis B serologies
> - Hepatitis C serologies
> - Lipid panel, fasting
>
> Age-appropriate cancer screening
>
> History, review of systems, and physical examination–driven laboratory and imaging studies
>
> *Abbreviation:* HIV, human immunodeficiency virus.

spongiotic dermatitis are common presentations of ICI dermatitis.[69] Psoriasiform, vitiliginous, and bullous dermatitis have also been reported. There have been at least 5 cases of GA

Table 3
Treatment options for granuloma annulare

Localized disease	Topical corticosteroids Intralesional corticosteroids Topical calcineurin inhibitors Cryosurgery Pulsed dye laser, Er:YAG laser, Nd:YAG laser, excimer laser
Widespread disease	Phototherapy • Narrowband UVB • UVA, PUVA • Photodynamic therapy Antibiotics • Tetracyclines • Rifampicin, ofloxacin, minocycline Immunomodulators • Dapsone • Fumaric acid esters • Antimalarials • Isotretinoin • Pentoxifylline Immunosuppressants • Cyclosporine • Methotrexate • TNF inhibitors

developing during therapy with ICIs.[70,71] An interesting corollary between the induction of GA after immune-checkpoint inhibition is prior reports of GA triggered by vaccination.[65,72–74] IFN-gamma has been found to play an important role and is a common denominator in ICI therapy as a possible biomarker for the overall response rate to anticancer immunotherapy,[75–77] vaccine efficacy,[78] and granuloma annulare.[67] It has been proposed that the IFN-gamma signal and strong Th1 cellular immunity induced by vaccines may lead to GA,[67,73] which may also be the case in checkpoint inhibitor–associated GA.

New Evidence-Based Treatment for Granuloma Annulare

In updates for treatment, Grewal and colleagues[79] performed a single-institution retrospective analysis of 35 patients with histologically confirmed GA and response to antimalarials. Within this cohort, 18 patients were treated with hydroxychloroquine, of which 10 (55.6%) improved. Six of those treatment-failure patients were then treated with chloroquine, of which 100% improved. The average duration with hydroxychloroquine and chloroquine before noting improvement was 3.6 and 3.0 months, respectively. These data suggest that antimalarials should be considered as a first-line treatment of generalized granuloma annulare.

REVIEW OF REACTIVE GRANULOMATOUS DERMATITIDES (PALISADED NEUTROPHILIC GRANULOMATOUS DERMATITIS AND INTERSTITIAL GRANULOMATOUS DERMATITIS)
Palisaded Neutrophilic Granulomatous Dermatitis

Epidemiology
Palisaded neutrophilic granulomatous dermatitis (PNGD) is a noninfectious granulomatous dermatitis that is thought to represent a reaction pattern seen in association with several systemic diseases. PNGD encompasses various terms, such as *Churg-Strauss granuloma*, *cutaneous extravascular necrotizing granuloma*, *rheumatoid papules*, *Winkelmann granuloma*, and *rheumatoid papules*. The complex and evolving nomenclature has made studying this entity very difficult. Therefore, not much is known about the epidemiology of PNGD. Although reports of PNGD in children are rare, the diseases can occur in patients of all ages. Females are affected more frequently than males in a ratio of approximately 3:1.[80] PNGD has many systemic associations, often rheumatologic in nature, which may help explain its increased incidence in females (**Box 3**). The strongest association between systemic disease and PNGD is connective tissue disease, followed by inflammatory arthritides and lymphoproliferative diseases. PNGD is also rarely associated with autoimmune disease, infection, and drugs.

Box 3
Diseases associated with palisaded neutrophilic and granulomatous dermatitis

Connective tissue disease
- Systemic lupus erythematosus
- Systemic sclerosis
- Undifferentiated connective tissue disease
- ANCA-associated vasculitis
- Erythema elevatum diutinum
- Sjogren syndrome
- Mixed cryoglobulinemia
- Takayasu aortitis

Inflammatory arthritides
- Rheumatoid arthritis
- Ankylosing spondylitis
- Juvenile idiopathic arthritis

Lymphoproliferative disease
- Acute myelogenous leukemia
- Chronic myelomonocytic leukemia
- Multiple myeloma
- Lymphoma

Other
- Sarcoidosis
- Ulcerative colitis
- Crohn disease
- Celiac disease and type I diabetes
- Behçet disease
- Multiple sclerosis
- Subacute bacterial endocarditis
- Hepatitis
- Streptococcal infection
- AIDS

Medications
- TNF inhibitors
- Allopurinol

Abbreviation: ANCA, antineutrophil cytoplasmic antibody.

Etiopathogenesis

The cause of PNGD is unknown. Given that PNGD typically occurs in association with systemic disease, it is supposed that it represents a reactive dermatitis secondary to internal inflammation.[81] Etiologic theories for PNGD include a delayed-type hypersensitivity reaction,[82] low-grade small-vessel vasculitis,[83,84] immune complex deposition,[83,85] and abnormal neutrophil activation.

Clinical and histologic presentation

PNGD is characterized by symmetric skin-colored to erythematous to hyperpigmented smooth, umbilicated, or crusted papules and plaques on the elbows and knees. However, many other clinical presentations and morphologies have been described, including urticarial or annular plaques,[86,87] erythematous nodules with and without scale,[86,88] papulonodules,[89] and linear bands.[80,86] Other distributions beyond elbows and hands have been described, including the legs,[82] nose,[90] cheek, and scalp.[80]

On histologic examination, a biopsy of PNGD can reveal a range of findings, which may vary with respect to the age of the lesion or possibly the underlying associated disease.[91] Ten percent to 30% of early lesions of PNGD reveal signs of frank leukocytoclastic vasculitis or features of intense neutrophilic inflammation and karyorrhectic debris.[83,86] In older lesions, there is degenerated collagen surrounded by palisading histiocytes and small granulomas and later areas of fibrosis.[86,91] Mucin is rare, potentially helping distinguish it from interstitial GA.

Review of Interstitial Granulomatous Dermatitis

Epidemiology

Interstitial granulomatous dermatitis (IGD) encompasses various entities, including IGD with arthritis, IGD with cords and arthritis, linear subcutaneous bands of rheumatoid arthritis, linear rheumatoid nodules, linear granuloma annulare, railway track dermatitis, and Ackerman syndrome. As with PNGD, the evolving nomenclature and taxonomy of IGD has made it difficult to study. As with PNGD, IGD is seen in all ages but less commonly reported in children[92]; the female to male ratio is similarly 3:1.[93] IGD has numerous systemic associations, many that overlap with those of PNGD. Of the associated diseases, inflammatory arthritides have the strongest association, followed by connective tissue diseases and hematologic disorders. IGD can also be associated with solid organ malignancies, autoimmune diseases, infections, and medications (**Box 4**). Interstitial granulomatous drug reaction (IGDR), initially described by Magro and colleagues,[94] is thought by some to represent a separate entity from IGD triggered by a drug. However, IGDR may represent a subtype if IGD associated with a drug.[81]

Etiopathogenesis

IGD is not well understood. It is thought to be a nonspecific sign of immune dysregulation or dysfunction, as it often occurs in association with systemic inflammation. It may be that immune complexes in dermal vessels leads to inflammation, damaged collagen, and subsequent granulomatous infiltrate,[95] which is similar to the proposed etiopathogenesis for PNGD. In IGDR, it was proposed that a drug trigger might alter the antigenicity of dermal collagen or perturb dermal collagen repair mechanisms.[94]

Clinical and histologic presentation

The initial description of IGD was linear subcutaneous cords on the proximal trunk[96]; however, that presentation may be uncommon and represents less than 10% of cases.[93] Lesions of IGD typically occur symmetrically on the lateral upper trunk, proximal inner arms, and proximal thighs but also the buttocks, abdomen, breast, and umbilicus. Other than linear rope-like lesions, IGD has been described as skin-colored to erythematous to violaceous patches or plaques in morphologies, including annular,[97] polycyclic,[98] cockades,[99] and atrophic hyperpigmented[100]; diffuse macular erythema[93]; subcutaneous nodules[101]; periungual and mucosal erythema[102]; and elbow papules and nodules (similar to those of PNGD).[103] The clinical manifestations of IGDR are often described as annular erythematous to violaceous plaques on the inner arms, proximal inner thighs, proximal trunk, and intertriginous sites.

Histologic evaluation of IGD reveals histiocytes scattered throughout the dermis, frequent palisading around foci of fragmented, and degenerated collagen, often leading to visible clefting called the "floating sign."[93] The histology of IGDR, in additional to interstitial histiocytes with granulomas and rare giant cells palisading around altered collagen, has some distinct features, including vacuolar interface dermatitis with dyskeratosis, lymphoid atypia, and prominent tissue eosinophilia.[94] Biopsies of IGD and IGDR are typically lacking vasculitis and mucin deposition, in contradistinction with PNGD and GA, respectively.

Box 4
Diseases associated with interstitial granulomatous dermatitis

Inflammatory arthritides
- Rheumatoid arthritis
- Seronegative inflammatory arthritis

Connective tissue disease
- Systemic lupus erythematosus
- Undifferentiated connective tissue disease

Hematologic disorders
- Immunoglobulin A gammopathy
- Anemia and thrombocytopenia
- Lymphoma
- Myelodysplastic syndrome
- Leukemia
- Multiple myeloma

Solid organ malignancies
- Breast
- Endometrial
- Lung
- Esophageal
- Prostate

Other
- Autoimmune hepatitis
- Primary biliary cirrhosis
- Uveitis
- Chronic inflammatory demyelinating polyneuropathy
- Autoimmune thyroiditis
- Antiphospholipid antibody syndrome
- Diabetes
- Vitiligo
- Pulmonary coccidioidomycosis
- Pulmonary silicosis
- *B burgdorferi* infection
- Hepatitis C and mixed cryoglobulinemia

Medications
- Tumor necrosis factor inhibitors
- Soy
- Angiotensin converting enzyme inhibitors
- Furosemide
- Quetiapine
- Talimogene laherparepvec

WHAT IS NEW IN PALISADING NEUTROPHILIC AND GRANULOMATOUS DERMATITIS AND INTERSTITIAL GRANULOMATOUS DERMATITIS

As described earlier, there is significant overlap in the risk factors, systemic associations, clinical description, and histologic findings of PNGD and IGD/IGDR (**Fig. 4**). Additionally, the ever-evolving nomenclature makes understanding the literature and studying these entities very difficult. In 2015, Rosenbach (author M.R.) and English[81] proposed an umbrella term called *reactive granulomatous dermatitis* to encompass the overlapping clinical and histologic entities of PNGD and IGD/IGDR. Although various distinct clinical and histologic patterns have been described (eg, linear cords in IGD or vasculitis and karyorrhexis in PNGD), these may represent distinction without difference. Considering many recent reports of difficult-to-classify granulomatous dermatitis seen in anticancer therapy, the umbrella term of *reactive granulomatous dermatitis* becomes even more useful.[104–107] Given the clinical and histologic overlap, the initial evaluation will largely be the same and the management directed at removing or treating the underlying cause of the reactive dermatitis. It may be helpful to further subcategorize reactive granulomatous dermatitis for the purposes of basic and translational research.

A summary of the initial evaluation and management of patients with reactive granulomatous dermatitis is described in **Table 4**.

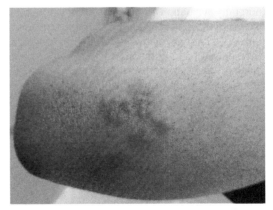

Fig. 4. Reactive granulomatous dermatitis (PNGD-like). Brown-pink indurated papules coalescing into a plaque on the elbow. On histology, there is exuberant interstitial granulomatous inflammation in areas arranged around small foci of altered collagen without mucin, eosinophils, neutrophils, lymphoid atypia, or vasculitis.

Table 4
Recommended evaluation and management for patients with reactive granulomatous dermatitis

Evaluate for drug-induced disease	Review of medications	• Prescription medications, over-the-counter medications, including supplements, herbal medications, dietary habits • Focus on calcium channel blockers, beta-blockers, angiotensin converting enzyme inhibitors, statins
Evaluate for systemic disease	Connective tissue disease	• Antinuclear antibodies • Antineutrophilic cytoplasmic antibodies • Additional testing dictated by systemic signs and symptoms
	Arthritis	• Rheumatoid factor, cyclic citrullinated peptide • Rheumatology evaluation • Consider imaging
	Malignancy	• Age-appropriate cancer screen • CBC with differential • Serum and urine protein electrophoresis with immunofixation electrophoresis
	Other	• Chest radiography • Occult infections (endocarditis, HIV, hepatitis, pulmonary fungal infection)
Management	General	• Skin biopsy • Medication cessation trial when indicated (at least 3 mo) • Control underlying systemic disease
	Reactive granulomatous dermatitis-specific treatment	• Watchful waiting • Topical or intralesional corticosteroids • NSAIDs • Dapsone • Hydroxychloroquine • Systemic corticosteroids • Consider additional agents in extensive/treatment-resistant cases

Abbreviations: CBC, complete blood count; HIV, human immunodeficiency virus; NSAIDs, nonsteroidal antiinflammatory drugs.

SUMMARY

Inflammatory granulomatous dermatitides are a poorly understood diverse group of disorders. Their management generally requires a thorough evaluation to identify underlying associated diseases or culprit triggers, including detailed history, review of systems, physical examination, in addition to laboratory and imaging investigation. High-quality data to inform clinical decision-making and treatment are lacking. Immunotherapy for the treatment of cancer is elucidating the mechanism for the etiopathogenesis and possible treatment approaches for inflammatory granulomatous dermatitides. Further research is needed in this domain.

REFERENCES

1. Ungprasert PWD, Crowson CS, Matteson EL. Epidemiology of cutaneous sarcoidosis, 1976-2013: a population-based study from Olmsted County, Minnesota. J Eur Acad Dermatol Venereol 2016;3:1799–804.

2. Baughman RP, Teirstein AS, Judson MA, et al. Clinical characteristics of patients in a case control study of sarcoidosis. Am J Respir Crit Care Med 2001;164(10 Pt 1):1885–9.

3. Goldstein RA, Janicki BW, Mirro J, et al. Cell-mediated immune responses in sarcoidosis. Am Rev Respir Dis 1978;117(1):55–62.

4. Bindoli S, Dagan A, Torres-Ruiz JJ, et al. Sarcoidosis and autoimmunity: from genetic background to environmental factors. Isr Med Assoc J 2016; 18(3–4):197–202.

5. Oswald-Richter KA, Beachboard DC, Seeley EH, et al. Dual analysis for mycobacteria and propionibacteria in sarcoidosis BAL. J Clin Immunol 2012; 32(5):1129–40.

6. Eishi Y. Etiologic aspect of sarcoidosis as an allergic endogenous infection caused by Propionibacterium acnes. Biomed Res Int 2013;2013: 935289.

7. Dubaniewicz A, Kampfer S, Singh M. Serum antimycobacterial heat shock proteins antibodies in sarcoidosis and tuberculosis. Tuberculosis 2006; 86(1):60–7.

8. Iannuzzi MC, Rybicki BA, Teirstein AS. Sarcoidosis. N Engl J Med 2007;357(21):2153–65.

9. Izbicki G, Chavko R, Banauch GI, et al. World Trade Center "sarcoid-like" granulomatous pulmonary disease in New York City Fire Department rescue workers. Chest 2007;131(5): 1414–23.

10. Sola R, Boj M, Hernandez-Flix S, et al. Silica in oral drugs as a possible sarcoidosis-inducing antigen. Lancet 2009;373(9679):1943–4.

11. Chen ES, Moller DR. Sarcoidosis–scientific progress and clinical challenges. Nat Rev Rheumatol 2011;7(8):457–67.

12. Sakthivel P, Bruder D. Mechanism of granuloma formation in sarcoidosis. Curr Opin Hematol 2017; 24(1):59–65.

13. Sahashi K, Ina Y, Takada K, et al. Significance of interleukin 6 in patients with sarcoidosis. Chest 1994;106(1):156–60.

14. Marcoval J, Mana J, Rubio M. Specific cutaneous lesions in patients with systemic sarcoidosis: relationship to severity and chronicity of disease. Clin Exp Dermatol 2011;36(7):739–44.

15. Milman N, Selroos O. Pulmonary sarcoidosis in the Nordic countries 1950-1982. II. Course and prognosis. Sarcoidosis 1990;7(2):113–8.

16. Mangas C, Fernandez-Figueras MT, Fite E, et al. Clinical spectrum and histological analysis of 32 cases of specific cutaneous sarcoidosis. J Cutan Pathol 2006;33(12):772–7.

17. Birnbaum MR, Ma MW, Fleisig S, et al. Nivolumab-related cutaneous sarcoidosis in a patient with lung adenocarcinoma. JAAD Case Rep 2017;3(3): 208–11.

18. Tetzlaff MT, Nelson KC, Diab A, et al. Granulomatous/sarcoid-like lesions associated with checkpoint inhibitors: a marker of therapy response in a subset of melanoma patients. J Immunother Cancer 2018;6(1):14.

19. Dimitriou F, Frauchiger AL, Urosevic-Maiwald M, et al. Sarcoid-like reactions in patients receiving modern melanoma treatment. Melanoma Res 2018;28(3):230–6.

20. Cotliar J, Querfeld C, Boswell WJ, et al. Pembrolizumab-associated sarcoidosis. JAAD Case Rep 2016;2(4):290–3.

21. Reddy SB, Possick JD, Kluger HM, et al. Sarcoidosis following anti-PD-1 and anti-CTLA-4 therapy for metastatic melanoma. J Immunother 2017; 40(8):307–11.

22. Chopra A, Nautiyal A, Kalkanis A, et al. Drug-induced sarcoidosis-like reactions. Chest 2018. https://doi.org/10.1016/j.chest.2018.03.056.

23. van de Schans SA, van Spronsen DJ, Hooijkaas H, et al. Excess of autoimmune and chronic inflammatory disorders in patients with lymphoma compared with all cancer patients: a cancer registry-based analysis in the south of the Netherlands. Autoimmun Rev 2011;10(4):228–34.

24. Arish N, Kuint R, Sapir E, et al. Characteristics of sarcoidosis in patients with previous malignancy: causality or coincidence? Respiration 2017;93(4): 247–52.

25. Brincker H, Wilbek E. The incidence of malignant tumours in patients with respiratory sarcoidosis. Br J Cancer 1974;29(3):247–51.

26. Le Jeune I, Gribbin J, West J, et al. The incidence of cancer in patients with idiopathic pulmonary fibrosis and sarcoidosis in the UK. Respir Med 2007;101(12):2534–40.

27. Seersholm N, Vestbo J, Viskum K. Risk of malignant neoplasms in patients with pulmonary sarcoidosis. Thorax 1997;52(10):892–4.

28. Ungprasert P, Crowson CS, Matteson EL. Risk of malignancy among patients with sarcoidosis: a population-based cohort study. Arthritis Care Res 2017;69(1):46–50.

29. El-Khalawany M, Mosbeh A, Aboeldahab S, et al. Cutaneous sarcoidosis: a new subset in the spectrum of paraneoplastic dermatoses. Clin Exp Dermatol 2018;43(6):683–91.

30. Cousin S, Toulmonde M, Kind M, et al. Pulmonary sarcoidosis induced by the anti-PD1 monoclonal antibody pembrolizumab. Ann Oncol 2016;27(6): 1178–9.

31. Papanikolaou IC, Sharma OP. The relationship between sarcoidosis and lymphoma. Eur Respir J 2010;36(5):1207–9.

32. London J, Grados A, Ferme C, et al. Sarcoidosis occurring after lymphoma: report of 14 patients and review of the literature. Medicine 2014; 93(21):e121.

33. Gaughan EM. Sarcoidosis, malignancy and immune checkpoint blockade. Immunotherapy 2017;9(13):1051–3.

34. Celada LJ, Rotsinger JE, Young A, et al. Programmed death-1 inhibition of phosphatidylinositol 3-kinase/AKT/mechanistic target of rapamycin signaling impairs sarcoidosis CD4(+) T cell proliferation. Am J Respir Cell Mol Biol 2017;56(1):74–82.

35. Xu J, Sun HH, Fletcher CD, et al. Expression of programmed cell death 1 ligands (PD-L1 and PD-L2) in histiocytic and dendritic cell disorders. Am J Surg Pathol 2016;40(4):443–53.

36. Braun NA, Celada LJ, Herazo-Maya JD, et al. Blockade of the programmed death-1 pathway restores sarcoidosis CD4(+) T-cell proliferative capacity. Am J Respir Crit Care Med 2014;190(5): 560–71.

37. Muller SA, Winkelmann RK. Necrobiosis lipoidica diabeticorum. A clinical and pathological investigation of 171 cases. Arch Dermatol 1966;93(3): 272–81.

38. Muller SA, Winkelmann RK. Necrobiosis lipoidica diabeticorum histopathologic study of 98 cases. Arch Dermatol 1966;94(1):1–10.

39. Erfurt-Berge C, Dissemond J, Schwede K, et al. Updated results of 100 patients on clinical features and therapeutic options in necrobiosis lipoidica in a retrospective multicentre study. Eur J Dermatol 2015;25(6):595–601.

40. O'Toole EA, Kennedy U, Nolan JJ, et al. Necrobiosis lipoidica: only a minority of patients have diabetes mellitus. Br J Dermatol 1999; 140(2):283–6.

41. Lowitt MH, Dover JS. Necrobiosis lipoidica. J Am Acad Dermatol 1991;25(5 Pt 1):735–48.

42. Peyri J, Moreno A, Marcoval J. Necrobiosis lipoidica. Semin Cutan Med Surg 2007;26(2):87–9.

43. Hammer E, Lilienthal E, Hofer SE, et al. Risk factors for necrobiosis lipoidica in Type 1 diabetes mellitus. Diabet Med 2017;34(1):86–92.

44. Engel MF, Smith JG Jr. The pathogenesis of necrobiosis lipoidica. Necrobiosis lipoidica, a form fruste of diabetes mellitus. Arch Dermatol 1960; 82:791–7.

45. Boateng B, Hiller D, Albrecht HP, et al. Cutaneous microcirculation in pretibial necrobiosis lipoidica. Comparative laser Doppler flowmetry and oxygen partial pressure determinations in patients and healthy probands. Hautarzt 1993;44(9):581–6 [in German].

46. Ngo B, Wigington G, Hayes K, et al. Skin blood flow in necrobiosis lipoidica diabeticorum. Int J Dermatol 2008;47(4):354–8.

47. Oikarinen A, Mortenhumer M, Kallioinen M, et al. Necrobiosis lipoidica: ultrastructural and biochemical demonstration of a collagen defect. J Invest Dermatol 1987;88(2):227–32.

48. Holland C, Givens V, Smoller BR. Expression of the human erythrocyte glucose transporter Glut-1 in areas of sclerotic collagen in necrobiosis lipoidica. J Cutan Pathol 2001;28(6):287–90.

49. Sparrow G, Abell E. Granuloma annulare and necrobiosis lipoidica treated by jet injector. Br J Dermatol 1975;93(1):85–9.

50. Wanat KRM. Necrobiosis lipoidica. In: Callen J, editor. UpToDate. Waltham (MA): UpToDate. Accessed May 29, 2018.

51. Basoulis D, Fragiadaki K, Tentolouris N, et al. Anti-TNFalpha treatment for recalcitrant ulcerative necrobiosis lipoidica diabeticorum: a case report and review of the literature. Metabolism 2016;65(4): 569–73.

52. Malemud CJ. The role of the JAK/STAT signal pathway in rheumatoid arthritis. Ther Adv Musculoskelet Dis 2018;10(5–6):117–27.

53. Damsky W, King BA. JAK inhibitors in dermatology: the promise of a new drug class. J Am Acad Dermatol 2017;76(4):736–44.

54. Heim MH. The Jak-STAT pathway: cytokine signalling from the receptor to the nucleus. J Recept Signal Transduct Res 1999;19(1–4):75–120.

55. Malemud CJ. Recent advances in neutralizing the IL-6 pathway in arthritis. Open access Rheumatol 2009;1:133–50.

56. Malemud CJ, Sun Y, Pearlman E, et al. Monosodium urate and tumor necrosis factor-alpha increase apoptosis in human chondrocyte cultures. Rheumatology (Sunnyvale) 2012;2:113.

57. Lee JJ, English JC 3rd. Improvement in ulcerative necrobiosis lipoidica after janus kinase-inhibitor therapy for polycythemia vera. JAMA Dermatol 2018;154(6):733–4.

58. Muhlbauer JE. Granuloma annulare. J Am Acad Dermatol 1980;3(3):217–30.

59. Piette EW, Rosenbach M. Granuloma annulare: clinical and histologic variants, epidemiology, and genetics. J Am Acad Dermatol 2016;75(3): 457–65.

60. Yun JH, Lee JY, Kim MK, et al. Clinical and pathological features of generalized granuloma annulare with their correlation: a retrospective multicenter study in Korea. Ann Dermatol 2009;21(2):113–9.

61. Keimig EL. Granuloma annulare. Dermatol Clin 2015;33(3):315–29.

62. Spring P, Vernez M, Maniu CM, et al. Localized interstitial granuloma annulare induced by subcutaneous injections for desensitization. Dermatol Online J 2013;19(6):18572.

63. Cassone G, Tumiati B. Granuloma annulare as a possible new adverse effect of topiramate. Int J Dermatol 2014;53(2):259–61.

64. Yoon NY, Lee NR, Choi EH. Generalized granuloma annulare after bacillus Calmette-Guerin vaccination, clinically resembling papular tuberculid. J Dermatol 2014;41(1):109–11.

65. Criado PR, de Oliveira Ramos R, Vasconcellos C, et al. Two case reports of cutaneous adverse reactions following hepatitis B vaccine: lichen planus and granuloma annulare. J Eur Acad Dermatol Venereol 2004;18(5):603–6.

66. Gass JK, Todd PM, Rytina E. Generalized granuloma annulare in a photosensitive distribution resolving with scarring and milia formation. Clin Exp Dermatol 2009;34(5):e53–5.

67. Fayyazi A, Schweyer S, Eichmeyer B, et al. Expression of IFNgamma, coexpression of TNFalpha and matrix metalloproteinases and apoptosis of T lymphocytes and macrophages in granuloma annulare. Arch Dermatol Res 2000;292(8):384–90.

68. Mempel M, Musette P, Flageul B, et al. T-cell receptor repertoire and cytokine pattern in granuloma annulare: defining a particular type of cutaneous granulomatous inflammation. J Invest Dermatol 2002;118(6):957–66.

69. Min Lee CK, Li S, Tran DC, et al. Characterization of dermatitis after PD-1/PD-L1 inhibitor therapy and association with multiple oncologic outcomes: a retrospective case-control study. J Am Acad

Dermatol 2018. https://doi.org/10.1016/j.jaad.2018. 05.035.

70. Wu J, Kwong BY, Martires KJ, et al. Granuloma annulare associated with immune checkpoint inhibitors. J Eur Acad Dermatol Venereol 2018;32(4): e124–6.

71. Charollais R, Aubin F, Roche-Kubler B, et al. Two cases of granuloma annulare under anti-PD1 therapy. Ann Dermatol Venereol 2018;145(2):116–9 [in French].

72. Kakurai M, Kiyosawa T, Ohtsuki M, et al. Multiple lesions of granuloma annulare following BCG vaccination: case report and review of the literature. Int J Dermatol 2001;40(9):579–81.

73. Nagase K, Koba S, Okawa T, et al. Generalized granuloma annulare following BCG vaccination, mimicking papular tuberculid. Eur J Dermatol 2011;21(6):1001–2.

74. Wolf F, Grezard P, Berard F, et al. Generalized granuloma annulare and hepatitis B vaccination. Eur J Dermatol 1998;8(6):435–6.

75. Remon J, Chaput N, Planchard D. Predictive biomarkers for programmed death-1/programmed death ligand immune checkpoint inhibitors in non-small cell lung cancer. Curr Opin Oncol 2016; 28(2):122–9.

76. McNamara MJ, Hilgart-Martiszus I, Barragan Echenique DM, et al. Interferon-gamma production by peripheral lymphocytes predicts survival of tumor-bearing mice receiving dual PD-1/CTLA-4 blockade. Cancer Immunol Res 2016;4(8):650–7.

77. Choueiri TK, Fishman MN, Escudier B, et al. Immunomodulatory activity of nivolumab in metastatic renal cell carcinoma. Clin Cancer Res 2016; 22(22):5461–71.

78. Ozgur A, Xiang Z, Radev DR, et al. Literature-based discovery of IFN-gamma and vaccine-mediated gene interaction networks. J Biomed Biotechnol 2010;2010:426479.

79. Grewal SK, Rubin C, Rosenbach M. Antimalarial therapy for granuloma annulare: results of a retrospective analysis. J Am Acad Dermatol 2017; 76(4):765–7.

80. Hantash BM, Chiang D, Kohler S, et al. Palisaded neutrophilic and granulomatous dermatitis associated with limited systemic sclerosis. J Am Acad Dermatol 2008;58(4):661–4.

81. Rosenbach M, English JC 3rd. Reactive granulomatous dermatitis: a review of palisaded neutrophilic and granulomatous dermatitis, interstitial granulomatous dermatitis, interstitial granulomatous drug reaction, and a proposed reclassification. Dermatol Clin 2015;33(3):373–87.

82. Kim SK, Park CK, Park YW, et al. Palisaded neutrophilic granulomatous dermatitis presenting as an unusual skin manifestation in a patient with Behcet's disease. Scand J Rheumatol 2005;34(4):324–7.

83. Finan MC, Winkelmann RK. The cutaneous extravascular necrotizing granuloma (Churg-Strauss granuloma) and systemic disease: a review of 27 cases. Medicine 1983;62(3):142–58.

84. Al-Daraji WI, Coulson IH, Howat AJ. Palisaded neutrophilic and granulomatous dermatitis. Clin Exp Dermatol 2005;30(5):578–9.

85. Misago N, Shinoda Y, Tago M, et al. Palisaded neutrophilic granulomatous dermatitis with leukocytoclastic vasculitis in a patient without any underlying systemic disease detected to date. J Cutan Pathol 2010;37(10):1092–7.

86. Sangueza OP, Caudell MD, Mengesha YM, et al. Palisaded neutrophilic granulomatous dermatitis in rheumatoid arthritis. J Am Acad Dermatol 2002;47(2):251–7.

87. Mahmoodi M, Ahmad A, Bansal C, et al. Palisaded neutrophilic and granulomatous dermatitis in association with sarcoidosis. J Cutan Pathol 2011;38(4): 365–8.

88. Asahina A, Fujita H, Fukunaga Y, et al. Early lesion of palisaded neutrophilic granulomatous dermatitis in ulcerative colitis. Eur J Dermatol 2007;17(3):234–7.

89. Muscardin LM, Cota C, Amorosi B, et al. Erythema elevatum diutinum in the spectrum of palisaded neutrophilic granulomatous dermatitis: description of a case with rheumatoid arthritis. J Eur Acad Dermatol Venereol 2007;21(1):104–5.

90. Collaris EJ, van Marion AM, Frank J, et al. Cutaneous granulomas in rheumatoid arthritis. Int J Dermatol 2007;46(Suppl 3):33–5.

91. Chu P, Connolly MK, LeBoit PE. The histopathologic spectrum of palisaded neutrophilic and granulomatous dermatitis in patients with collagen vascular disease. Arch Dermatol 1994;130(10): 1278–83.

92. Moon HR, Lee JH, Won CH, et al. A child with interstitial granulomatous dermatitis and juvenile idiopathic arthritis. Pediatr Dermatol 2013;30(6):e272–3.

93. Peroni A, Colato C, Schena D, et al. Interstitial granulomatous dermatitis: a distinct entity with characteristic histological and clinical pattern. Br J Dermatol 2012;166(4):775–83.

94. Magro CM, Crowson AN, Schapiro BL. The interstitial granulomatous drug reaction: a distinctive clinical and pathological entity. J Cutan Pathol 1998; 25(2):72–8.

95. Tomasini C, Pippione M. Interstitial granulomatous dermatitis with plaques. J Am Acad Dermatol 2002;46(6):892–9.

96. Dykman CJ, Galens GJ, Good AE. Linear subcutaneous bands in rheumatoid arthritis. an unusual form of rheumatoid granuloma. Ann Intern Med 1965;63:134–40.

97. Zoli A, Massi G, Pinnelli M, et al. Interstitial granulomatous dermatitis in rheumatoid arthritis responsive to etanercept. Clin Rheumatol 2010;29(1):99–101.

98. Felcht M, Faulhaber J, Gottmann U, et al. Interstitial granulomatous dermatitis (Ackerman's Syndrome). Eur J Dermatol 2010;20(5):661–2.

99. Blaise S, Salameire D, Carpentier PH. Interstitial granulomatous dermatitis: a misdiagnosed cutaneous form of systemic lupus erythematosus? Clin Exp Dermatol 2008;33(6):712–4.

100. Jabbari A, Cheung W, Kamino H, et al. Interstitial granulomatous dermatitis with arthritis. Dermatol Online J 2009;15(8):22.

101. Busquets-Perez N, Narvaez J, Valverde-Garcia J. Interstitial granulomatous dermatitis with arthritis (Ackerman syndrome). J Rheumatol 2006;33(6):1207–9.

102. Nakamura N, Asai J, Daito J, et al. Interstitial granulomatous dermatitis? An unusual presentation in the mucosa and periungual skin. J Dermatol 2011;38(4):382–5.

103. Lee KJ, Lee ES, Lee DY, et al. Interstitial granulomatous dermatitis associated with autoimmune hepatitis. J Eur Acad Dermatol Venereol 2007;21(5):684–5.

104. Jansen YJ, Janssens P, Hoorens A, et al. Granulomatous nephritis and dermatitis in a patient with BRAF V600E mutant metastatic melanoma treated with dabrafenib and trametinib. Melanoma Res 2015;25(6):550–4.

105. Kubicki SL, Welborn ME, Garg N, et al. Granulomatous dermatitis associated with ipilimumab therapy (ipilimumab associated granulomatous dermatitis). J Cutan Pathol 2018;45(8):636–8.

106. Trinidad C, Nelson KC, Glitza Oliva IC, et al. Dermatologic toxicity from immune checkpoint blockade therapy with an interstitial granulomatous pattern. J Cutan Pathol 2018;45(7):504–7.

107. Everett AS, Pavlidakey PG, Contreras CM, et al. Chronic granulomatous dermatitis induced by talimogene laherparepvec therapy of melanoma metastases. J Cutan Pathol 2018;45(1):48–53.

Comorbidities in Dermatology
What's Real and What's Not

Azam Qureshi, BA[a], Adam Friedman, MD[a,b],*

KEYWORDS

- Atopic dermatitis • Lymphoma • Hidradenitis suppurativa • Alopecia areata • Thyroid disease
- Chronic urticaria • Pemphigus

KEY POINTS

- Evidence suggests an association between atopic dermatitis and lymphoma, whereas an association with pancreatic cancer is more equivocal.
- Recent literature highlights the following: (1) patients with hidradenitis suppurativa bear a significant burden of psychiatric disease; (2) thyroid disease is the most common autoimmune comorbidity affecting patients with alopecia areata; (3) chronic urticaria has been shown to be associated with increased prevalence of various inflammatory diseases.
- A recent association between pemphigus and chronic obstructive pulmonary disorder warrants further investigation to determine clinical relevance.
- Further studies are needed to investigate causal inferences that possibly contribute to associations highlighted within the article.

INTRODUCTION

Comorbidities in dermatologic disease have been found to cover a diverse array of body systems from cardiovascular to psychiatric, thereby conferring a variable and multifaceted impact on patients.[1,2] Several highly prevalent dermatologic diseases carry a strong burden of comorbidities, underscoring their relevance to both patients and providers.[1,3–5] Whether comorbid conditions are causal of the dermatologic disease in question, are an effect of the disease, or share a common pathophysiologic underpinning are all questions requiring investigation beyond epidemiologic study. Nonetheless, identification and understanding of comorbidities are important goals and serve to provide practitioners with a context of how best to evaluate patients. Improved context of evaluation can enhance the provider's ability to recommend screening and preventive measures.[6] Understanding of comorbidities is of significant importance for treatment algorithms, because they can influence treatment choice and may lead to the identification of novel therapeutic targets through elucidating common underlying pathophysiologic mechanisms.

In terms of comorbidities, several dermatologic diseases extensively studied include acne, psoriasis, and rosacea.[1,4,5] This present article, however, seeks to highlight newer associations drawn from the current literature studying diseases that have emerging work in the area of comorbidities. Specifically, this review focuses on several dermatologic diseases including atopic dermatitis (AD),

Disclosures: Neither author has any relevant financial conflicts of interest.
[a] Department of Dermatology, George Washington Medical Faculty Associates, 2150 Pennsylvania Avenue Northwest, Suite 2B-427, Washington, DC 20037, USA; [b] Department of Dermatology, George Washington School of Medicine and Health Sciences, 2150 Pennsylvania Avenue Northwest, Suite 2B-427, Washington, DC 20037, USA
* Corresponding author. Department of Dermatology, George Washington School of Medicine and Health Sciences, 2150 Pennsylvania Avenue Northwest, Suite 2B-427, Washington, DC, 20037.
E-mail address: ajfriedman@mfa.gwu.edu

Dermatol Clin 37 (2019) 65–71
https://doi.org/10.1016/j.det.2018.07.007
0733-8635/19/© 2018 Elsevier Inc. All rights reserved.

derm.theclinics.com

hidradenitis suppurativa (HS), alopecia areata (AA), chronic urticaria (CU), and members of the pemphigus family. Selected comorbidities with each disease are discussed and evaluated in regard to supporting evidence in the literature.

CONTENT

Atopic Dermatitis and Cancer (Lymphoma and Pancreatic)

AD is a chronic inflammatory skin disease affecting 10% to 20% of individuals from industrialized countries with onset usually occurring in childhood.[7] Aside from the classic triad including allergic rhinitis and asthma, evidence for several different AD comorbidities have surfaced in the literature, including autoimmune, neuropsychiatric, and cardiovascular diseases, as well as with certain cancers.[7] Recent studies providing evidence for neoplastic comorbidities with AD have implicated both lymphoma and pancreatic cancer, raising questions regarding the strength of these associations, their clinical relevance, and explanations for the co-occurences.[8,9]

Recent results from a large cross-sectional study comparing more than 8000 Danish subjects with AD with more than 40,000 control subjects provide evidence supporting an association of AD with lymphoma and pancreatic cancer.[10] Of these cancers for which AD subjects were found to be at significantly increased risk, the odds ratio (OR) (adjusted for sex, age, socioeconomic status [SES], and number of clinic visits) was highest (2.91, 95% confidence interval [CI]: 1.50–5.66, P = .0016) for patients developing pancreatic cancer.[10] Patients were also found to be at significantly increased risk for nonmelanoma skin cancer (OR: 2.07, 95% CI: 1.67–2.55, $P<.0001$) and lymphoma (OR: 1.86, 95% CI: 1.43–2.40, $P<.0001$).[10] Hagströmer and colleagues[11] found a standardized incidence ratio of 1.9 (95% CI: 1.0–3.4) for patients with AD with pancreatic cancer in a retrospective cohort study of more than 15,000 inpatients, which also demonstrated increases in cancers of the esophagus, lung, and brain in patients with AD. Despite these data, evidence associating pancreatic cancer with AD is inconsistent overall, as several case-control studies have demonstrated an opposite trend (decreased incidence of pancreatic cancer) in patients with AD, albeit with smaller sample sizes.[9,12–15] Systematic reviews and meta-analyses investigating the risk of pancreatic cancer in AD are lacking.

Association of AD with lymphoma, however, has a stronger level of support in the literature. In a study population consisting of 4,518,131 patients in the United Kingdom, Arana and colleagues[16] conveyed a greater incidence of lymphoma in patients with AD (2.05 cases per 10,000 person-years, 95% CI: 1.49–2.75) in comparison to patients without AD (1.69 cases per 10,000 person-years, 95% CI: 1.65–1.74) (statistical significance not presented). AD association with lymphoma has also been supported by a recent meta-analysis carried out by Legendre and colleagues.[8] They found that patients with AD described by the 5 cohort studies included had a significant relative risk of 1.43 (95% CI 1.12–1.81) for developing lymphoma overall.[8] In 18 case-control studies included, the investigators noted no significantly increased risk of lymphoma.[8] Studies, overall, provided evidence that worse AD severity is associated with lymphoma development, a finding that may be attributable to an increased use of high-potency topical corticosteroids and topical calcineurin inhibitors.[8] Other possible explanations include the use of systemic immunosuppressive therapeutic agents and diagnostic overlap of AD with cutaneous T-cell lymphoma in certain cases.[7,10,17] AD association with cancer may also be explained by chronic immune system stimulation by antigen, which may trigger increased random prooncogenic mutations.[18]

Although AD associations with both pancreatic cancer and lymphoma warrant attention and further investigation, the association with lymphoma is currently better supported in the literature than the association with pancreatic cancer. Despite strong evidence attributing AD with increased risk of lymphoma, a relative risk of 1.43 offered by the meta-analysis conducted by Legendre and colleagues[8] suggest a low level of association with clinical relevance yet to be determined.

Hidradenitis Suppurativa and Psychiatric Disorders

HS is a chronic inflammatory condition involving recurring inflammatory abscesslike nodules that can evolve into scars and draining sinuses located in the intertriginous skin of the axillary and inguinal regions.[19,20] Evidence suggests disease prevalence rates range from 0.5% to 4%, with a significant burden of comorbidity including arthropathies, dyslipidemia, and polycystic ovarian syndrome.[19,21,22] The psychiatric comorbidities of HS, in particular, have been the subject of increasing investigation in recent years.[20,23–25]

A recently published retrospective study investigating psychiatric disorders in patients with HS conveyed these patients suffer from mental disorders more than patients with psoriasis, a dermatologic disease well known for psychiatric comorbidities.[23,26] Psychiatric disorders were noted in a surprising 24.1% of the 4337 HS patient sample.[23] Furthermore, psychotic disorders were noted in 4.7% of patients.[23] Schizophrenia and bipolar disorder, specifically, were noted to occur with increased prevalence in HS patients (with ORs, 95% CIs of 1.57, 1.24–1.98 and 1.81, 1.47–2.23, respectively).[23] The burden of psychiatric comorbidity in HS was recently investigated in children, as well, in a Finnish retrospective case-control study with findings recently published in the *Journal of the American Academy of Dermatology*.[25] The investigators found that children younger than 18 years old with HS were at increased risk for psychiatric disorders in comparison to control children with benign melanocytic nevi (OR: 3.31, 95% CI: 1.86–5.90) (*P*-value not presented).[25]

Depression, specifically, has been the subject of recent literature regarding comorbidities in HS.[20,24] Onderdijk and colleagues[24] found that mean Major Depression Inventory (MDI) scores were higher in 211 patients with HS (11.0) in comparison to 233 control outpatient dermatology patients with other diseases (7.2, *P*<.0001). Furthermore, a significantly higher proportion of patients with HS (21%, 44/211) received MDI scores that indicate possible depression in comparison to control patients (11%, 26/233, *P* = .006).[24] Although MDI scores did not correlate significantly with Hurley stage, they did produce significant and positive correlations with frequency of flares, pain and itch symptoms, and sick days due to HS.[24] Findings from this study were confirmed by another report published 2 years later, which detailed results from a cross-sectional study of 3207 HS patients and 6412 gender- and age-matched control patients who were members of the largest managed care organization in Israel.[20] Investigators found a significantly increased prevalence of diagnosed depression in patients with HS (5.9%) in comparison to patients without HS (3.5%, *P*<.001).[20] Patients with HS also received significantly more anxiety diagnoses (3.9%) in comparison to control patients (2.4%, *P*<.001).[20]

Explanations for the association of HS with depression and anxiety may be in part due to the impaired quality of life accompanying HS.[27,28] Furthermore, proinflammatory cytokines, including TNFα and IL-1, have been shown to be elevated in patients with both psychiatric disorders as well as lesional HS skin.[29–31] These common inflammatory mediators may provide evidence for a common underlying pathophysiologic mechanism. Most importantly, however, these associations underscore the importance of a multidisciplinary approach to caring for a patient with HS, with particular attention for patient's mental health.

Alopecia Areata and Other Autoimmune Diseases

AA is a form of nonscarring hair loss with a strong autoimmune component.[6] Because AA can affect up to 1% to 2% of the US population, it is vital to understand its comorbidities, which include associations with other autoimmune-mediated diseases.[6,32,33] A recent retrospective study conducted by Magen and colleagues[34] quantified a significantly elevated OR for patients with AA developing systemic autoimmune disease (4.72, 3.99–5.57, *P*<.001) in comparison to age- and gender-matched controls. Although autoimmune disease associations with AA are well characterized in the literature, an emerging emphasis on thyroid disease has conveyed its relatively high prevalence and clinical relevance.[6,35]

Multiple studies provide evidence that thyroid disease is the most commonly occurring autoimmune comorbidity in patients with AA.[35,36] In an 11-year retrospective review of 3568 AA patients in Boston, Massachusetts, investigators found that thyroid disease was the most prevalent autoimmune comorbidity (14.6%), followed by diabetes mellitus (11.1%), psoriasis/psoriatic arthritis (6.3%), systemic lupus erythematosus (SLE) (4.3%), RA (3.9%), and inflammatory bowel disease (2.0%).[35] Although this study lacked a control comparator group, a controlled, retrospective review was published several years later by Conic and colleagues.[36] They conveyed that thyroid disease was the only autoimmune disorder occurring significantly more frequently in 584 patients with AA (18.80%) in comparison to age-matched control patients without AA (7.56%, *P*<.001, OR: 2.84, 95% CI: 1.55–5.18).[36] Notably, diabetes mellitus, psoriasis, RA, and SLE prevalence was not statistically different between groups.[36]

Thyroid disease in relation to age of onset has also been evaluated in patients with AA. Because of the growing body of evidence supporting a substantial prevalence of thyroid disorders in patients with AA, Patel and colleagues[6] sought to determine criteria for thyroid function screening in children. From the data generated by their retrospective review, investigators concluded that routine thyroid function screening should be considered specifically in AA patients with a history of Down syndrome, atopy, or a family history of thyroid disease.[6] Furthermore, pediatric AA patients with clinical findings that suggest thyroid dysfunction should also be advised to undergo testing.[6] In a study conducted by Lee and colleagues[37] comparing comorbidities between those with early onset AA (before age 13) versus late-onset AA (all other AA patients), investigators determined that thyroid disease was the most common comorbidity noted in patients with late-onset disease and that it affected a significantly higher percentage of patients in comparison to the early onset group (12.2% vs 0.0%, P<.001). This comparison is limited by the relatively low sample of early onset patients (N = 98) in comparison to late-onset patients (N = 773).[37] Nonetheless, these data supporting the prevalence of thyroid disorders in patients with late-onset disease underscore the importance of defining consensus guidelines for thyroid disease screening in patients with late-onset AA as well.

Chronic Urticaria and Chronic Inflammatory Diseases

CU is a condition involving at least 6 weeks of pruritic hives and/or angioedema occurring on a repeated basis.[38] Prevalence rates of disease have ranged from 0.6% to 0.8% in European populations.[39,40] Recent studies have linked CU with various inflammatory diseases including peptic ulcer, hepatitis B or C, periodontitis, and AA.[34,38]

In the aforementioned study conducted by Magen and colleagues,[34] patients with AA were found to have a significantly elevated OR for chronic spontaneous urticaria (6.15, 4.06–9.32, P<.001) in comparison to age- and gender-matched controls. A recent study also demonstrated a coincidence of autoimmune disease in pediatric patients with CU (6/139 children) while noting a 17% prevalence of autoimmune disease in family members of children with CU.[41] This study, however, was limited in its lack of a control group.[41] A recent Taiwanese study also studied comorbidities in patients with CU in comparison to the normal population.[38] Patients with CU demonstrated significantly higher risk for chronic inflammatory diseases in comparison to normal patients, with a standardized prevalence ratio of 1.57 (95% CI: 1.56–1.58).[38] Overall, the prevalence of inflammatory diseases was 9.78% in patients with CU, and inflammatory diseases were the most common comorbidity overall.[38] Peptic ulcer accounted for most diagnoses (4.83%), followed by periodontitis (2.82%) and hepatitis B or C (1.64%).[38] Standardized prevalence ratios in comparison to the normal population ranged from 1.29 to 1.76 for all individual inflammatory diseases observed, including chronic sinusitis, otitis media, periodontitis, diverticulitis, Helicobacter pylori infection, peptic ulcer, and hepatitis B or C.[38]

The abundant evidence supporting an association between inflammatory diseases and chronic urticaria, along with the observed increased prevalence of inflammatory disease increasing with longer persisting chronic urticaria, supports the hypothesis that persistence of disease may be encouraged by chronic inflammation.[38] Furthermore, nonsteroidal anti-inflammatory agents and antibiotics taken by these patients may play a role in inducing chronic urticaria in some cases.[38]

Pemphigus and Lung Disease

Pemphigus is a family of autoimmune diseases involving cutaneous vesiculobullous lesions. Although rare, patients suffer from painful blisters and an increased mortality rate that can be improved with treatment.[42–44] In addition to well-characterized autoimmune disease associations, lung diseases, including bronchiolitis obliterans (BO) and chronic obstructive pulmonary disease (COPD), have been shown to be associated with various forms of pemphigus.[45–47]

BO, an airway disease involving inflammation and scarring, is well known as a comorbidity affecting 6% to 25% of patients with paraneoplastic pemphigus (PNP), a form of pemphigus usually associated with lymphoproliferative disorders.[46–48] Approximately 30% of mortality in PNP is due to progressive respiratory failure, with BO or BO-type features.[49] Recent work has proposed that the pathogenesis of BO association with PNP is possibly related to an autoantigen of epiplakin, which is a member of the plakin family of cytoplasmic proteins.[47,50] Plakin proteins may be found in respiratory epithelium and have been implicated in being autoimmune targets in PNP along with desmoglein proteins.[49]

A recent cross-sectional study conveyed results showing a higher prevalence of COPD in patients with pemphigus (13.4%) in comparison to age-, sex-, and ethnicity-matched subjects in a control group (10.1%, P<.001).[45] Importantly, although this study found a significant risk of COPD in patients with pemphigus (OR: 1.3, 95% CI:1.1–1.5, P = .001), there was no similar increased risk of lung cancer in patients with pemphigus after controlling for confounding variables including SES, smoking, and health care utilization.[45] Smoking was less prevalent in the pemphigus patient group in comparison to the control group.[45] Furthermore, the observed association was weaker amongst smokers in each group and statistical significance remained after adjustment for smoking.[45]

Association of pemphigus with COPD has been hypothesized to be due to a possible autoimmune contribution to development of COPD, as suggested by several studies conveying an increased risk for developing COPD in patients with autoimmune disease.[45,51–54] Respiratory epithelium is not known to express desmogleins 1 and 3, which are targets of autoimmunity in pemphigus foliaceus and vulgaris, respectively.[45,55] Previous work, however, has both provided evidence for autoimmune comorbidity in patients with COPD without history of smoking, while suggesting an autoimmune contribution to COPD possibly by way of circulating antibodies against elastin.[45,52,56] The pathophysiologic basis of pemphigus and other autoimmune comorbidities in COPD is not well understood. Further investigation is needed to better characterize the risk and clinical relevance of COPD in dermatologic patients with pemphigus and other autoimmune diseases.

SUMMARY

This article highlights recent developments in the literature regarding comorbidities in several dermatologic diseases. Some comorbidities investigated have a strong body of supporting evidence, including AD and lymphoma, HS and psychiatric disease, AA and thyroid disease, and CU and chronic inflammatory diseases.[8,10,16,19,20,24,25,34–36,38] These findings have begun to shape expert opinions on practice of care, as thyroid disease screening guidelines in children with AA have emerged recently.[6] Other associations suggested by recent literature have more equivocal records of evidence, including AD and pancreatic cancer.[10–15] Furthermore, additional investigation is needed to better elucidate the clinical relevance of a recently determined slight, but significant, increased risk of COPD in patients with pemphigus.[45]

The literature, overall, is somewhat limited in that most studies are epidemiologic in nature and therefore present correlative associations without evidence of causation. Furthermore, interpretations of results should be handled cautiously, because statistical significance is not always a marker for clinical relevance. Although ORs may present a convincing level of risk, the absolute risks may still be exceedingly low for rare comorbidities.

Understanding comorbidities in dermatologic disease is highly relevant to providers for the purposes of not only screening but also patient counseling and disease prevention. Elucidation of these comorbidities can also shed light on common underlying pathophysiologic mechanisms that guide the treatment decisions and development of future potential therapeutic targets. Future studies in this area should seek to investigate a basis for causal inference for observed comorbidities while generating further evidence-based screening guidelines for comorbidities in dermatologic patients.

REFERENCES

1. Oliveira M de F, Rocha B de O, Duarte GV. Psoriasis: classical and emerging comorbidities. An Bras Dermatol 2015;90(1):9–20.

2. Pompili M, Innamorati M, Trovarelli S, et al. Suicide risk and psychiatric comorbidity in patients with psoriasis. J Int Med Res 2016;44(1 Suppl):61–6.

3. Wilmer EN, Gustafson CJ, Davis SA, et al. Most common dermatologic conditions encountered by dermatologists and nondermatologists. Cutis 2014; 94(6):285–92.

4. Silverberg JI, Silverberg NB. Epidemiology and extracutaneous comorbidities of severe acne in adolescence: a U.S. population-based study. Br J Dermatol 2014;170(5):1136–42.

5. Vera N, Patel NU, Seminario-Vidal L. Rosacea comorbidities. Dermatol Clin 2018;36(2):115–22.

6. Patel D, Li P, Bauer AJ, et al. Screening guidelines for thyroid function in children with alopecia areata. JAMA Dermatol 2017;153(12):1307–10.

7. Andersen YMF, Egeberg A, Skov L, et al. Comorbidities of atopic dermatitis: beyond rhinitis and asthma. Curr Dermatol Rep 2017;6(1):35–41.

8. Legendre L, Barnetche T, Mazereeuw-Hautier J, et al. Risk of lymphoma in patients with atopic dermatitis and the role of topical treatment: a systematic review and meta-analysis. J Am Acad Dermatol 2015;72(6):992–1002.

9. Wang H, Diepgen TL. Atopic dermatitis and cancer risk. Br J Dermatol 2006;154(2):205–10.

10. Ruff S, Egeberg A, Andersen Y, et al. Prevalence of cancer in adult patients with atopic dermatitis: a nationwide study. Acta Derm Venereol 2017;97(9): 1127–9.

11. Hagströmer L, Ye W, Nyrén O, et al. Incidence of cancer among patients with atopic dermatitis. Arch Dermatol 2005;141(9):1123–7.

12. Mack TM, Yu MC, Hanisch R, et al. Pancreas cancer and smoking, beverage consumption, and past medical history. J Natl Cancer Inst 1986;76(1): 49–60. Available at: http://www.ncbi.nlm.nih.gov/pubmed/3455742. Accessed June 6, 2018.

13. Bueno de Mesquita HB, Maisonneuve P, Moerman CJ, et al. Aspects of medical history and exocrine carcinoma of the pancreas: a population-based case-control study in The Netherlands. Int J Cancer 1992;52(1):17–23. Available at: http://www.ncbi.nlm.nih.gov/pubmed/1500222. Accessed June 6, 2018.

14. Jain M, Howe GR, St Louis P, et al. Coffee and alcohol as determinants of risk of pancreas cancer: a case-control study from Toronto. Int J Cancer 1991;47(3): 384–9. Available at: http://www.ncbi.nlm.nih.gov/pubmed/1993545. Accessed June 6, 2018.

15. Holly EA, Eberle CA, Bracci PM. Prior history of allergies and pancreatic cancer in the san francisco bay area. Am J Epidemiol 2003;158(5):432–41.

16. Arana A, Wentworth CE, Fernández-Vidaurre C, et al. Incidence of cancer in the general population and in patients with or without atopic dermatitis in the U.K. Br J Dermatol 2010;163(5):1036–43.

17. Miyagaki T, Sugaya M. Erythrodermic cutaneous T-cell lymphoma: how to differentiate this rare disease from atopic dermatitis. J Dermatol Sci 2011;64(1):1–6.

18. Holly EA, Bracci PM. Population-based study of non-Hodgkin lymphoma, histology, and medical history among human immunodeficiency virus-negative participants in San Francisco. Am J Epidemiol 2003;158(4):316–27.

19. Shlyankevich J, Chen AJ, Kim GE, et al. Hidradenitis suppurativa is a systemic disease with substantial comorbidity burden: a chart-verified case-control analysis. J Am Acad Dermatol 2014;71(6):1144–50.

20. Shavit E, Dreiher J, Freud T, et al. Psychiatric comorbidities in 3207 patients with hidradenitis suppurativa. J Eur Acad Dermatol Venereol 2015;29(2):371–6.

21. Jemec GB, Heidenheim M, Nielsen NH. The prevalence of hidradenitis suppurativa and its potential precursor lesions. J Am Acad Dermatol 1996;35(2 Pt 1):191–4. Available at: http://www.ncbi.nlm.nih.gov/pubmed/8708018. Accessed June 12, 2018.

22. Cosmatos I, Matcho A, Weinstein R, et al. Analysis of patient claims data to determine the prevalence of hidradenitis suppurativa in the United States. J Am Acad Dermatol 2013;69(5):819.

23. Huilaja L, Tiri H, Jokelainen J, et al. Patients with hidradenitis suppurativa have a high psychiatric disease burden: a Finnish Nationwide Registry Study. J Invest Dermatol 2018;138(1):46–51.

24. Onderdijk AJ, van der Zee HH, Esmann S, et al. Depression in patients with hidradenitis suppurativa. J Eur Acad Dermatol Venereol 2013;27(4):473–8.

25. Tiri H, Jokelainen J, Timonen M, et al. Somatic and psychiatric comorbidities of hidradenitis suppurativa in children and adolescents. J Am Acad Dermatol 2018. https://doi.org/10.1016/j.jaad.2018.02.067.

26. Ferreira BI, Abreu JL, Dos Reis JP, et al. Psoriasis and associated psychiatric disorders: a systematic review on etiopathogenesis and clinical correlation. J Clin Aesthet Dermatol 2016;9(6):36–43. Available at: http://jcadonline.epubxp.com/t/9606-journal-of-clinical-and-aesthetic-dermatology%5Cnhttp://ovidsp.ovid.com/ovidweb.cgi?T=JS&PAGE=reference&D=emedx&NEWS=N&AN=20160476754.

27. Alavi A, Farzanfar D, Lee RK, et al. The contribution of malodour in quality of life of patients with hidradenitis suppurativa. J Cutan Med Surg 2018;22(2):166–74.

28. Kluger N, Ranta M, Serlachius M. The burden of hidradenitis suppurativa in a cohort of patients in southern finland: a pilot study. Skin Appendage Disord 2017;3(1):20–7.

29. Henje Blom E, Lekander M, Ingvar M, et al. Pro-inflammatory cytokines are elevated in adolescent females with emotional disorders not treated with SSRIs. J Affect Disord 2012;136(3):716–23.

30. Lee S-Y, Chen S-L, Chang Y-H, et al. Inflammation's association with metabolic profiles before and after a twelve-week clinical trial in drug-naïve patients with bipolar ii disorder. PLoS One 2013;8(6):e66847.

31. van der Zee HH, de Ruiter L, van den Broecke DG, et al. Elevated levels of tumour necrosis factor (TNF)-α, interleukin (IL)-1β and IL-10 in hidradenitis suppurativa skin: a rationale for targeting TNF-α and IL-1β. Br J Dermatol 2011;164(6):1292–8.

32. Safavi KH, Muller SA, Suman VJ, et al. Incidence of alopecia areata in olmsted county, minnesota, 1975 through 1989. Mayo Clin Proc 1995;70(7):628–33.

33. Wasserman D, Guzman-Sanchez DA, Scott K, et al. Alopecia areata. Int J Dermatol 2007;46(2):121–31.

34. Magen E, Chikovani T, Waitman D-A, et al. Association of alopecia areata with atopic dermatitis and chronic spontaneous urticaria. Allergy Asthma Proc 2018;39(2). https://doi.org/10.2500/aap.2018.39.4114.

35. Huang KP, Mullangi S, Guo Y, et al. Autoimmune, atopic, and mental health comorbid conditions associated with alopecia areata in the United States. JAMA Dermatol 2013;149(7):789–94.

36. Conic RZ, Miller R, Piliang M, et al. Comorbidities in patients with alopecia areata. J Am Acad Dermatol 2017;76(4):755–7.

37. Lee NR, Kim B-K, Yoon NY, et al. Differences in comorbidity profiles between early-onset and late-onset alopecia areata patients: a retrospective study of 871 Korean patients. Ann Dermatol 2014;26(6):722–6.

38. Chu C-Y, Cho Y-T, Jiang J-H, et al. Epidemiology and comorbidities of patients with chronic urticaria in Taiwan: a nationwide population-based study. J Dermatol Sci 2017;88(2):192–8.

39. Zuberbier T, Balke M, Worm M, et al. Epidemiology of urticaria: a representative cross-sectional population survey. Clin Exp Dermatol 2010;35(8):869–73.

40. Gaig P, Olona M, Muñoz Lejarazu D, et al. Epidemiology of urticaria in Spain. J Investig Allergol Clin Immunol 2004;14(3):214–20. Available at: http://www.ncbi.nlm.nih.gov/pubmed/15552715. Accessed June 12, 2018.

41. Netchiporouk E, Sasseville D, Moreau L, et al. Evaluating comorbidities, natural history, and predictors of early resolution in a cohort of children with chronic urticaria. JAMA Dermatol 2017;153(12):1236–42.

42. Huang Y-H, Kuo C-F, Chen Y-H, et al. Incidence, mortality, and causes of death of patients with pemphigus in Taiwan: a nationwide population-based study. J Invest Dermatol 2012;132(1):92–7.

43. Kridin K, Sagi S, Bergman R. Mortality and cause of death in israeli patients with pemphigus. Acta Derm Venereol 2017;97(5):607–11.

44. Langan SM, Smeeth L, Hubbard R, et al. Bullous pemphigoid and pemphigus vulgaris - Incidence and mortality in the UK: population based cohort study. Br Med J 2008;337(7662):160–3.

45. Kridin K, Comaneshter D, Batat E, et al. COPD and lung cancer in patients with pemphigus- a population based study. Respir Med 2018;136:93–7.

46. Lee S, Yamauchi T, Ishii N, et al. Achievement of the longest survival of paraneoplastic pemphigus with bronchiolitis obliterans associated with follicular lymphoma using R-CHOP chemotherapy. Int J Hematol 2017;106(6):852–9.

47. Tsuchisaka A, Numata S, Teye K, et al. Epiplakin is a paraneoplastic pemphigus autoantigen and related to bronchiolitis obliterans in Japanese patients. J Invest Dermatol 2016;136(2):399–408.

48. Leger S, Picard D, Ingen-Housz-Oro S, et al. Prognostic factors of paraneoplastic pemphigus. Arch Dermatol 2012;148(10):1165.

49. Nousari HC, Deterding R, Wojtczack H, et al. The mechanism of respiratory failure in paraneoplastic pemphigus. N Engl J Med 1999;340(18):1406–10.

50. Takahashi M, Shimatsu Y, Kazama T, et al. Paraneoplastic pemphigus associated with bronchiolitis obliterans. Chest 2000;117(2):603–7. Available at: http://www.ncbi.nlm.nih.gov/pubmed/10669715. Accessed June 13, 2018.

51. Cosio MG, Saetta M, Agusti A. Immunologic aspects of chronic obstructive pulmonary disease. N Engl J Med 2009;360(23):2445–54.

52. Birring SS, Brightling CE, Bradding P, et al. Clinical, radiologic, and induced sputum features of chronic obstructive pulmonary disease in nonsmokers: a descriptive study. Am J Respir Crit Care Med 2002;166(8):1078–83.

53. Birring SS, Morgan AJ, Prudon B, et al. Respiratory symptoms in patients with treated hypothyroidism and inflammatory bowel disease. Thorax 2003;58(6):533–6.

54. Hemminki K, Liu X, Ji J, et al. Subsequent COPD and lung cancer in patients with autoimmune disease. Eur Respir J 2011;37(2):463–5.

55. Nguyen VT, Ndoye A, Bassler KD, et al. Classification, clinical manifestations, and immunopathological mechanisms of the epithelial variant of paraneoplastic autoimmune multiorgan syndrome: a reappraisal of paraneoplastic pemphigus. Arch Dermatol 2001;137(2):193–206.

56. Lee SH, Goswami S, Grudo A, et al. Antielastin autoimmunity in tobacco smoking-induced emphysema. Nat Med 2007;13(5):567–9.

Updates in Melanoma

Elisabeth Hamelin Tracey, MD, Alok Vij, MD*

KEYWORDS

- Melanoma • Skin cancer • Melanoma staging • Gene expression profiling • Immunotherapy
- Targeted therapy for melanoma

KEY POINTS

- The incidence of melanoma and nonmelanoma skin cancers is increasing rapidly in the United States, as is the understanding of the pathophysiology of melanoma.
- Recent revisions to the American Joint Committee on Cancer (AJCC) staging criteria incorporated evidence-based changes to better risk-stratify patients into similar prognostic groups.
- Promising tests are available to help stratify patients who may be at higher risk for disease recurrence or distant metastasis; however, the implementation and interpretation of these tests are still evolving.
- Targeted therapy and immunotherapies for advanced melanoma offer hope of a cure to patients who previously had a bleak prognosis.

Skin cancer in the United States has reached epidemic proportions. More than 5 million cases of skin cancer will be diagnosed in the United States this year. Nonmelanoma skin cancer (NMSC), comprising mostly basal cell carcinoma (BCC) and squamous cell carcinoma (SCC), is the most common type of malignancy in humans. Melanoma, less common but more aggressive than BCC and SCC, ranks as the sixth most common cancer in the United States and accounts for 1 death per hour.[1]

The incidence of NMSC is staggering, having increased 77% between 1994 and 2014, related to an aging population and increased emphasis on prompt diagnosis and treatment. The incidence of melanoma is also skyrocketing, and mortality is higher with melanoma compared with BCC and SCC. Cure rates for localized primary cutaneous melanoma are excellent if caught early and treated appropriately; however, metastatic spread to lymph nodes or distant sites is associated with much higher risk of death.[2]

In the past decade, the understanding of melanoma has shifted dramatically. The molecular pathogenesis of the disease has become increasingly clear: not only the mutations that allow for tumorigenesis but also the interactions with the immune system that allow tumor survival and distant metastasis. As a result, the diagnostic work-up, risk stratification, and treatment of melanoma are changing more rapidly than ever before.

Specifically, the American Joint Committee on Cancer (AJCC) staging system has been revised, incorporating evidence-based changes to better stratify patients into risk categories, improving prognostic accuracy. Sentinel lymph node biopsy (SLNB), standard of care for many patients with invasive melanoma, and completion lymph node dissection remain controversial because of conflicting results from prominent trials. SLNB can increase rates of cure for patients with evidence of advanced melanoma; however, many patients who die from melanoma have a negative SLNB; completion lymph node dissection was not superior to nodal observation in patients with nodal micrometastasis identified by SLNB. New molecular-based tests may be able to additionally stratify certain patients into more specific risk groups than SLNB alone; however, the literature related to the implementation and interpretation

Disclosure: Dr E.H. Tracey and Dr A. Vij have no disclosures related to this article.
Department of Dermatology, Dermatology and Plastic Surgery Institute, Cleveland Clinic Foundation, 9500 Euclid Avenue, Desk A61, Cleveland, OH 44195, USA
* Corresponding author.
E-mail address: vija@ccf.org

Dermatol Clin 37 (2019) 73–82
https://doi.org/10.1016/j.det.2018.08.003
0733-8635/19/© 2018 Elsevier Inc. All rights reserved.

of these studies is still evolving. In addition, the medications approved and under investigation to treat advanced melanoma are bringing hope (and cures) to patients who previously faced a bleak prognosis.

PATHOPHYSIOLOGY

Ultraviolet (UV) irradiation from sun exposure or indoor tanning bed use is the undisputed primary cause of cutaneous melanoma in sun-sensitive individuals.[3,4] The UV radiation induces a multitude of genetic changes in melanocytes, which can undergo malignant transformation as a result.

Genetic studies reveal approximately half of familial melanomas and one-quarter of sporadic melanomas may be caused by mutations in the tumor suppressor protein p16. Familial melanomas make up approximately 8% to 12% of all melanomas. Linkage studies have identified chromosome 9p21 as the familial melanoma gene locus.[5] Within the 9p21 region, specific mutations in the gene CDKN2A have been shown in familial melanoma kindreds. The CDKN2A gene is complex and codes for the p16 and p14arf proteins, both of which function to suppress cellular growth. Intact p16 inhibits cyclin-dependent kinases, a critical class of enzymes whose function is to promote cellular proliferation by inhibiting the retinoblastoma protein. Therefore, intact p16 is essential to arrest the cell cycle; mutations in p16 allow for continuous, unregulated cell division. In addition, the p14(ARF) protein may be important in enhancing the effect of another tumor suppressor, p53.[5]

Other critically important molecular signaling pathways in the development of melanoma are the mitogen-activated protein kinase (MAPK) and phosphatidylinositol-4,5-bisphosphate 3-kinase–protein kinase B (PI3K-AKT) pathways. Discovery of several abnormal variants in this pathway responsible for tumorigenesis, including the BRAF gene product, has allowed the development of targeted therapies for advanced melanoma. Among sporadic melanomas, almost half have mutations in the BRAF gene, including a common point mutation encoding for an altered protein, BRAFV600E. The MEK gene product, 1 step down the pathway from BRAF, can become altered in sporadic melanoma, as well as tumors that are resistant to targeted BRAF inhibition.

Mutations in c-KIT, a receptor tyrosine kinase involved in initiating the pathway, are rare overall but can be seen in certain types of the melanoma: acral melanoma; mucosal melanoma; and melanoma arising in areas of intermittent, intense sun exposure. Activating mutations at any point in the MAPK and PI3K-AKT pathways result in increased cellular proliferation and survival advantages of tumor cells.[6]

STAGING AND PROGNOSIS

Determining melanoma stage is important for planning appropriate treatment and assessing prognosis. The AJCC TNM (tumor, lymph node, metastasis) staging system breaks down the T classification based on the Breslow thickness; ulceration is classified as a high-risk feature for all tumors, and mitoses per square millimeter is a high-risk feature for tumors with a thickness less than 1 mm.[7]

Approximately 85% of patients with melanoma have localized disease (stages I and II) at presentation, about 15% have regional nodal disease, and only about 2% have distant metastases at the time of diagnosis.[1,2,8] Many factors affect the prognosis for stage I and II melanoma. Clinical factors associated with a favorable prognosis include younger age, female sex, and extremity lesions. Increasing Breslow thickness is the most important negative prognostic indicator, with worse survival for every stratum of tumor thickness in the AJCC staging guidelines. Other histologic variables associated with a poor prognosis include ulceration, diminished lymphoid response, evidence of tumor regression, microscopic satellites, lymphovascular invasion, and non–spindle-cell-type tumors.[9]

The presence of regional lymph node metastases imparts an overall 5-year melanoma-specific survival rate of 77% and a 10-year melanoma-specific survival of 69%. When adjusting for size of lymph node deposits and number of nodes involved, the melanoma-specific survival ranges from 57% to 82% at 5 years and 47% to 75% at 10 years.[7] The most important prognostic factor for stage III melanoma is the number of positive lymph nodes. Patients with nodal micrometastases have an improved survival compared with patients with clinically palpable nodes. Patients with melanoma on an extremity and younger age at diagnosis have been shown to have a better prognosis. If there are distant metastases, median survival is about 6 to 9 months.[1,2,7,8,10] For stage IV, the prognostic variables suggesting worse prognosis include increasing number of metastatic sites, visceral location of metastases (lung, liver, brain, bone), absence of resectable metastases, male sex, and shorter duration of remission.[1,2,7,8,10] Patients with nonvisceral disease (eg, skin, subcutaneous tissue, lymph nodes) have a better median survival rate, ranging from

12 to 15 months, and are more likely to respond to chemotherapy.[10]

In order to offer the best counseling to patients, all data related to the tumor must be synthesized into as precise a stage as possible. The revised TNM staging as proposed by the AJCC is presented at https://cancerstaging.org/.[7]

All data related to the tumor can be used to group patients into one of several clinical stages, as shown at https://cancerstaging.org/.[7] Clinical staging includes histologic data related to the primary tumor in addition to information from the clinical and radiologic evaluation for metastatic disease. Conventionally, clinical staging should be used after biopsy of the primary tumor, with clinical assessment for regional and distant metastases. As such, there is only 1 clinical stage for lymph node metastases and 1 stage for distant metastases. Pathologic assessment of the primary melanoma is used for both clinical and pathologic classification. A diagnostic evaluation of regional and distant metastases is included. Pathologic staging includes histologic information related to the primary tumor from biopsy and excision, and information about the regional lymph nodes after SLNB or completion lymph node dissection for clinically evident regional lymph node disease.

The prognosis for patients with localized primary cutaneous melanoma is mainly related to tumor thickness. Survival data for patients with nodal status known to be negative are shown at https://cancerstaging.org/.[7]

Prognosis for patients with nodal disease relates to the thickness of the primary tumor, the size and extent of metastatic deposits within the lymph node, and presence of distant metastases. The 5-year and 10-year survival data for patients with known metastatic disease in the lymph node are presented at https://cancerstaging.org/.[7]

Melanoma-specific survival data, when combining staging data for the primary tumor, nodal disease, and the presence or absence of distant metastases, are presented at https://cancerstaging.org/.[7]

Sentinel Lymph Node Biopsy

SLNB is a diagnostic and potentially therapeutic procedure to determine the presence or absence of metastatic melanoma cells in the draining nodal basin by removing the node that first receives and processes lymphatic fluid from the affected skin. Initially, lymphoscintigraphy is used to precisely map the draining nodal basin. A 1% isosulfan blue dye is injected around the cutaneous lesion to allow intraoperative localization of this sentinel lymph node. Alternately, a radioactive tracer

(technetium-99) can be injected at the lesion site. A gamma probe is used to pinpoint the radiolabeled lymph node, which is then removed for histopathologic review.[11]

Determination of the status of the sentinel lymph node is relevant for several reasons. Sentinel node biopsy is a fairly low-risk procedure that can help identify high-risk patients who may benefit from additional therapy, such as selective complete lymphadenectomy or adjuvant therapy with a targeted therapy, immunotherapy, or radiation therapy. It also provides a psychological benefit for patients whose biopsies do not reveal metastasis. In addition, the procedure may be associated with improved survival.[12]

National Comprehensive Cancer Network (NCCN) guidelines state that SLNB is important for staging but it has not been shown to improve rates of disease-specific survival in all patients. There has been 1 major randomized controlled trial evaluating the potential survival benefit of SLNB, the Multicenter Selective Lymphadenectomy Trial 1 (MSLT-1). Subset analysis of prospectively collected data from MSLT-1 suggests that a negative SLNB is associated with improvement in the distant metastasis-free survival rate in patients with melanomas 1.2 to 3.5 mm thick, compared with patients with melanomas of similar thickness who are initially observed and subsequently develop clinical nodal metastasis.[13]

The MSLT-1 did not find a statistically significant melanoma-specific survival difference for patients who underwent SLNB compared with those who were observed, which was the primary end point of the study. However, SLNB was associated with a longer disease-free survival (DFS) compared with observation.[13] The findings from MSLT-1, in addition to several previous studies, caused SLNB to become standard of care for melanoma. However, SLNB remains controversial because many patients with thin melanoma were excluded from MSLT-1 and a large proportion of patients with negative SLNB develop metastatic disease.

Only approximately one-third of patients who develop metastatic disease are identified at the time of diagnosis via SLNB.[9] In a large, single-institution survey, when lesions were stratified by Breslow thickness, no survival difference was found for patients with a negative biopsy compared with those with a positive biopsy. Lymph node status also did not show independent prognostic ability compared with Breslow thickness alone in multivariate analysis. However, the study was limited by a long period under review, spanning several eras of melanoma treatment; inability to control for adjuvant treatment; and a short follow-up time.[14–17]

SLNB is generally not recommended for in situ tumors or for stage I tumors with Breslow thickness less than or equal to 0.75 mm. Risk factors, when present, that may guide clinicians to consider SLNB on a patient-specific basis include ulceration, mitotic features, and lymphovascular invasion. These findings are uncommon in lesions less than or equal to 0.75 mm thick. For tumors with a Breslow thickness 0.76 to 1 mm without ulceration and with no mitoses per square millimeter, the NCCN guidelines recommend discussing and considering SLNB. For patients with clinically negative nodes with a primary tumor 0.76 to 1 mm thick with ulceration or any mitoses square millimeter or a tumor thicker than 1 mm, biopsy should be discussed and offered. SLNB is controversial for patients with Breslow thickness greater than 4 mm because of the poor prognosis associated with advancing tumor thickness. Despite the controversy, SLNB remains standard of care for these patients.[9]

Completion Lymph Node Dissection

Completion lymph node dissection is defined as removing regional lymph nodes that drain the site of the primary melanoma in the presence of nodal metastases, including sentinel lymph node positivity, ultrasonographic findings, or clinically palpable disease. Completion lymph node dissection for nodal micrometastatic disease detected by positive SLNB is a much-debated topic in the management of melanoma. The results of the Multicenter Selective Lymphadenectomy Trial II showed immediate completion lymph node dissection after positive SLNB was not superior to observation with routine nodal ultrasonography and delayed completion lymph node dissection in improving melanoma-specific survival rates, although there was increased disease control in the regional nodes and, thus, an improvement in DFS.[18]

The German Dermatologic Cooperative Oncology Group (DeCOG) study also attempted to clarify the impact of completion lymph node dissection in patients with positive SLNB. The trial was closed early because of difficulty enrolling patients; of the 1269 patients eligible for the trial with positive SLNB, only 473 (37%) were randomized. The DECOG-SLT trial revealed no survival benefit in patients treated with completion lymph node dissection compared with observation alone. The trial had short follow-up, median 35 months, but noted 3-year distant metastasis-free survival of 77% in the observation group compared with 74.9% in the treatment group. Although the trial was underpowered, the investigators recommend against completion lymph node dissection for patients with positive SLNB with metastatic deposits less than 1 mm in diameter.[19]

The Sunbelt Melanoma Trial attempted to clarify the role of high-dose interferon in patients with histologically positive SLNB in addition to the role of completion lymph node dissection in patients with histologically negative SLNB but evidence of nodal micrometastasis found by polymerase chain reaction (PCR). The trial did not find high-dose interferon improved disease-free survival or overall survival for patients with a single tumor-positive SLNB, although patient accrual goals were not met. Subgroup analysis suggested completion lymph node dissection may improve DFS, particularly at 5 years, without an impact on overall survival.[20]

Treatment should be tailored to the individual because patient-specific factors may warrant completion lymphadenectomy after a positive biopsy. Specifically, high-risk features include many of the exclusion criteria of the trial: extracapsular extension noted on SLNB, microsatellitosis of the primary tumor, greater than 3 involved nodes, greater than 2 involved nodal basins, and immunosuppression of the patient.[21]

MOLECULAR TESTING

Given the controversies surrounding SLNB and completion lymph node dissection, many clinicians have been searching for additional tests to identify patients at high risk for local recurrence, lymph node disease, or distant metastasis. Gene expression profiling has been used to further stratify patients with localized, node-negative disease into high-risk and low-risk categories for the development of metastatic disease.[22]

DecisionDx-Melanoma is a gene expression profile (GEP) test developed by Castle Biosciences, which measures expression levels of 28 discriminating genes and 3 control genes in tumor tissue of primary melanoma. Based on its genetic signature, a tumor is categorized in a binary system as either low risk (class I) or high risk (class II) for metastasis.

The purpose of development of this tool was to add prognostic value for patients with stage I and II melanoma, a group that has a heterogeneous disease course not precisely predicted with current staging methods.[23] Although there is some evidence that the test could contribute independent prognostic information to standard risk stratification methods, the data are mixed, and tangible improvement in clinical management has not been shown. Published studies to date have received funding from Castle Biosciences or were coauthored by individuals with disclosed affiliations with the company, with the exception of 1 independent study, which is explicitly identified later.

Development of the Gene Expression Profile

Gene selection
Most of the GEP panel was selected from genes in the published literature that consistently showed differing levels of expression in primary and metastatic melanoma tissue. Two gene probes were added for the 3′ and 5′ ends of the BRCA1-associated protein 1 transcript because of the significance of this gene in uveal and cutaneous melanoma. The remainder of the distinguishing genes as well as the control genes were selected from an existing uveal melanoma GEP after performing the test on metastatic and nonmetastatic cutaneous melanomas.

Development of the gene expression profile classification system
Reverse transcription PCR was performed on 107 stage I and II tumors from 3 institutions to determine expression levels of the selected genes. A radial basis machine predictive model was developed that generates a quantitative linear probability score from 0.0 to 1.0. Using a score cutoff of 0.5, the model divides tumors using a binary system of either low risk (class I) or high risk (class II) for metastasis. All of the 20 tumors in the development cohort that developed metastases were designated class II (100% sensitivity), whereas specificity of the model in the initial cohort was 78%.

Validation of the gene expression profile
The resulting GEP was validated with a unique cohort of 104 cases. DFS rates based on Kaplan-Meier analysis were 97% for class I and 31% for class 2 (P<.0001), similar to the results for the initial development cohort (100% for class 1 and 38% for class 2, P<.0001). After narrowing analysis to only stage I and II patients in the validation cohort with at least 5 years of follow-up or a metastatic event, significant stratification was seen between GEP classes for the end points of DFS, distant metastasis-free survival (DMFS), melanoma-specific survival, and overall survival. Multivariate Cox regression analysis of this subset revealed the GEP predicted metastatic risk independent of AJCC stage and individual patient-specific and tumor-specific factors of Breslow thickness, ulceration, mitotic rate, and age.[23]

MOLECULAR TESTING
Assessment of Prognostic Value

In a unique cohort of 523 patients, multivariate analysis revealed that class 2 status was an independent predictor of decreased recurrence-free survival (RFS) and DMFS. When evaluated by stage, RFS was significantly different between GEP classes in each of AJCC stages I to III. However, significant difference in DMFS was only shown in stage II and III patients and was not seen in stage I patients.[24]

Gene expression profile combined with an online prediction tool
The value of combining the GEP with an online prediction tool was analyzed in patients with stage I and II melanoma. The online tool (AJCC Individualized Melanoma Patient Outcome Prediction Tool), which is distinct from the AJCC staging system, generates a risk score on a continuum, but the investigators simplified results into a binary system for analysis. Combination of the 2 tests increased sensitivity for recurrence, distant metastasis, and death but also decreased specificity for each outcome. Although the investigators conclude that "gains in sensitivity when combining the GEP with AJCC tools outweigh the reduction in specificity,"[25] it should be noted that the optimized balance between sensitivity and specificity for any test is context specific and not absolute.

Further limitations of this study are characteristics of the study cohort. Median thickness of these stage I and stage II tumors was 1.5 mm, whereas median thickness of all invasive melanomas in the Surveillance, Epidemiology, and End Results (SEER) 9 registries during this time was 0.58 to 0.62 mm.[26] Results in this high-risk population may not be generalizable. In addition, most of the patients in this cohort were also in the original development cohort that the GEP test algorithm was designed to model, which diminishes the chances of the GEP accurately predicting their outcomes.[27]

Gene expression profile and sentinel lymph node biopsy
A retrospective analysis of the GEP was performed in 217 patients with patients with melanoma from 7 centers who had undergone SLNB and had at least 5 years of follow-up or a documented metastatic event. For each end point, DFS, DMFS, and overall survival, class 2 GEP signature had a higher hazard ratio than did positive SLNB. Multivariate regression analysis showed both SLNB and GEP as statistically significant predictors of DFS and DMFS, but only GEP predicted overall survival.

Combining GEP and SLNB led to identification of a group with the lowest risk (GEP class I, SLNB negative) with improved prediction of DFS, DMFS, and overall survival compared with either test alone. The 42% of patients who were classified as class II with a negative SLNB did not significantly differ from class II patients with a positive SLNB for any end point. Thus, the investigators suggest that a clinical application of the test would be to identify the SLNB-negative patients who are at high risk for metastasis.[28]

A major limitation of this study is that the cohort was not representative of the normal population of patients with melanoma. Only 21% of patients were AJCC stage I compared with about 40% in the general population, and only 17% of tumors were less than or equal to 1 mm thick compared with more than 60% in the general population.[29]

MOLECULAR TESTING
Independent Study of the Gene Expression Profile

Greenhaw and colleagues[30] analyzed the GEP in a cohort of 256 patients in an independent, non–industry-sponsored study. Overall, the test showed a 77% sensitivity and 87% specificity. Eighty-six percent of the tumors tested were stage I and the only tumor in that group that metastasized was GEP class 1. Twelve of the 37 stage II tumors metastasized, and the rate of metastasis in this group was 42% and 15% for class 2 and class 1 tumors, respectively. A limitation of this study is that median follow-up time was less than 2 years, and this study diverged from other studies in that it did not consider a positive SLNB a metastatic event.

Prospective Data

The first prospective study of the GEP, partially funded by Castle Biosciences, is underway, and interim results were published in 2017 with a median follow-up of 1.5 years in event-free patients. GEP independently predicted melanoma recurrence ($P<.01$) in multivariate Cox regression analysis but it did not independently predict distant metastasis or overall survival. Tumor thickness was the only variable found to be a significant predictor of distant metastasis and overall survival in this cohort.[31]

MOLECULAR TESTING
Clinical Significance

There are no established guidelines that recommend clinical situations in which to order GEP testing or changes in management based on GEP results. Studies to date of the clinical impact of the GEP assess actual or hypothetical management changes but do not assess tangible clinical outcomes.

Management changes

One prospective study of 156 patients at 6 institutions found documented management changes, which included frequency of examinations, recommendations for imaging, and referrals, after receipt of test results in 37% and 77% of class 1 and 2 patients, respectively. This study provides evidence that clinicians were significantly influenced by GEP results in the context of a prospective, industry-sponsored study of the impact of the test, but it is unclear whether the results are generalizable or whether the management changes were beneficial to the patients.[32]

A retrospective review of 91 patients with melanoma assessing the impact of GEP results on plans for multidisciplinary follow-up found that stage I and II patients designated as GEP class 1 were more likely to follow up with dermatology alone, whereas those designated as GEP class 2 were more likely to follow up with surgical oncology plus or minus a recommendation for adjuvant trial. No class 2 patients were advised to follow up with dermatology alone. Follow-up data are not available for assessment of whether more aggressive management affected outcomes or was an effective use of health care resources.[22]

In a survey performed following a presentation on the GEP, dermatology residents responded that they would alter clinical decisions such as the Breslow thickness at which to recommend SLNB, imaging, and oncology referral based on GEP results. The correlation between hypothetical decision making by trainees after a presentation on the GEP and actual management decisions by practicing dermatologists is unknown. Again, there is a lack of data to suggest what management changes, if any, would be appropriate in the proposed situations based on the additional data provided by GEP.[33]

When to order the gene expression profile test

The GEP test is commercially available but there is no consensus on an appropriate clinical situation for it to be ordered or offered to a patient. Svoboda and colleagues[34] performed an industry-sponsored survey of dermatologists and trainees at a national conference to determine how different clinical factors could influence ordering patterns. Tumor thickness greater than 0.5 mm, ulceration, and SLNB status were found to be influential. However, use of the GEP by these individual clinicians, one-third of whom were not previously familiar with the test, does not indicate appropriate use of the test.

The development of the GEP is part of a broader effort to improve the precision of melanoma risk stratification in order to provide better risk-appropriate care to patients with melanoma. Although there is evidence that the GEP yields prognostic information, the available data do not yet clearly support that it adds meaningful prognostic value beyond already-accepted risk stratification systems. Further prospective and independent studies will help define the utility of the GEP and clarify whether there are clinical situations in which the GEP would add value to patient care.

TARGETED THERAPIES FOR ADVANCED MELANOMA

Some of the most exciting breakthroughs in all of medicine relate to the interdisciplinary advances in the understanding of melanoma tumor biology and antitumor immunology over the past decade. These breakthroughs have translated into rapid advances in the treatment of advanced melanoma.[35] Historically, treatment options for metastatic melanoma have offered only incremental improvements in survival on the scale of months. The new generation of treatments has offered patients with metastatic melanoma the chance for durable DFS and, in some cases, a cure. In addition, patients with localized melanoma who are at high risk of developing metastatic disease may be treated with these newer agents.

BRAF Inhibitors

As discussed earlier, activating mutations in *BRAF* are common in melanoma. Two agents, vemurafenib and dabrafenib, are approved by the US Food and Drug Administration (FDA) for the treatment of tumors with the characteristic V600E mutation. Both vemurafenib and dabrafenib have been shown to provide significant improvements in progression-free survival compared with the traditional standard chemotherapy, dacarbazine. Treatment with vemurafenib was associated with a statistically significant improvement in overall survival; a trend to increased overall survival was identified with dabrafenib treatment, but the trend was not statistically significant.[36,37]

However, the discovery that most patients treated with single-agent BRAF inhibitors eventually have disease progression has tempered the initial optimism about these medications. Consequently, multiagent treatment strategies combining BRAF inhibition with another targeted treatment have largely replaced single-agent regimens in clinical practice.

MEK Inhibitors

After single-agent BRAF inhibition, multiple mutations can develop within tumors to reactivate the aberrant MAP kinase pathway, thus leading to treatment resistance and disease progression. Several substitution mutations in MEK1 have been identified that confer a survival advantage to tumor cells.

Trametinib is an FDA-approved MEK inhibitor that is indicated for single-agent therapy for advanced melanoma; additionally, cobimetinib has been approved for use in combination with vemurafenib for patients with a BRAF V600E mutation. Compared with standard chemotherapy, trametinib significantly lengthened both progression-free survival and overall survival.[38] Combination cobimetinib-vemurafenib therapy lengthened progression-free survival and median survival compared with chemotherapy.[39]

Combination BRAF-MEK inhibition was studied as adjuvant therapy for melanoma. Concurrent dabrafenib-trametinib therapy in patients with BRAF-mutant stage III melanoma reduced the risk of disease recurrence or death by 53% compared with placebo after 3 years. Preliminary data revealed an increased rate of overall survival: 77% in the placebo arm compared with 86% in the treatment arm.[40] As a result of the study, dabrafenib-trametinib was approved as an adjuvant treatment of patients with BRAF V600E-positive or V600K-positive melanoma.

NRAS Inhibitors

In addition to MEK1, *NRAS* gene mutations were also discovered in patients who developed resistance to single-agent BRAF inhibitors. Binimetinib is a MEK inhibitor that has activity against melanoma with a mutation in *NRAS*. At the time of this writing, it is still in clinical trials and has not been approved for use outside a clinical trial setting.

cKIT Inhibitors

cKIT gene mutations are infrequently identified in patients with acral, mucosal, or cutaneous melanoma in the setting of chronic sun damage. KIT inhibitors, including imatinib and nilotinib, have been studied more in patients with mucosal melanoma than primary cutaneous melanoma. Small trials have not shown KIT inhibitors to be significantly effective in melanoma; however, a subset of patients with mutations in exon 11 or 13 of the *KIT* gene more favorably respond to KIT inhibitors.[41,42] At the time of this writing, no KIT inhibitors have been approved for patients outside a clinical trial setting.

IMMUNOTHERAPIES FOR ADVANCED MELANOMA

Rapid advances in the understanding of melanoma tumor biology translated into the rapid deployment of targeted therapies against melanoma; at the same time, steady progress has been made in tumor-related immunology. Specifically, the discovery of immune checkpoints, considered the breakthrough of the year in 2013,[43] has led to the development of several drugs approved for patients with stage III or IV melanoma. Immune checkpoint inhibitors unleash the host's antitumoral immunity by preventing tumor cells from inactivating T cells via either cytotoxic T-lymphocyte antigen 4 (CTLA-4) or programmed cell death receptor 1 (PD-1).

Cytotoxic T-lymphocyte Antigen 4 Inhibitors

Ipilimumab was one of the first-approved immunotherapies for melanoma. Ipilimumab has shown prolonged overall survival in large clinical trials, with a prolonged survival benefit for those patients who respond well to treatment. In patients with metastatic melanoma who were not treated with other agents, ipilimumab plus dacarbazine increased overall survival compared with treatment with placebo plus dacarbazine. In addition, treatment with ipilimumab significantly increased overall survival and objective response rate in patients previously treated with chemotherapy or interleukin-2.[44] Across all trials, the minority of patients who have a complete response seem to have a durable survival: 22% of patients who were followed for at least 3 years survived and 21% survived to 10 years.[45]

Ipilimumab is approved for adjuvant therapy after surgical excision of high-risk melanomas. However, ipilimumab has become a second-line agent for adjuvant therapy for high-risk melanoma as well as primary immunotherapy for metastatic melanoma because of the improved efficacy and increased tolerability of PD-1 inhibitors.

Programmed Cell Death Receptor 1 Inhibitors

Pembrolizumab was compared with chemotherapy in patients refractory to ipilimumab in the KEYNOTE 002 study. In this pivotal study, patients treated with pembrolizumab had longer progression-free survival as well as a higher objective response rate compared with patients treated with chemotherapy.[46] In addition, in the KEYNOTE 006 trial, compared with ipilimumab treatment, pembrolizumab resulted in significantly improved progression-free survival, overall survival, and objective response rate.[47]

Nivolumab has been proved to be effective as monotherapy and in combination with the CTLA-4 inhibitor ipilimumab. In the CheckMate 066 trial, nivolumab was compared with dacarbazine in treatment-naive patients. Nivolumab was associated with significantly improved overall survival, progression-free survival, and objective response rate.[48] Nivolumab was also compared with chemotherapy in the CheckMate 037 trial for patients previously treated with ipilimumab and a BRAF inhibitor. Overall survival rates were not significantly different; however, objective responses were more common and the median duration of response was longer in patients treated with nivolumab.[49]

Ipilimumab and nivolumab were studied together against either ipilimumab or nivolumab in the 3-armed CheckMate 067 trial. Combination therapy with both ipilimumab and nivolumab was associated with improved progression-free survival, overall survival, and objective response rate compared with ipilimumab alone. However, the trial did not have suitable power to compare the combination treatment against nivolumab alone.[50] Nivolumab is also approved for adjuvant therapy and for treatment of patients with stage III melanoma.

SUMMARY

The landscape of melanoma diagnosis, staging and prognosis, and treatment has been fundamentally altered in the past decade. Updated data from previous iterations of the AJCC staging criteria allow more accurate prognosis. Further results from large clinical trials have not removed the controversy from SLNB and completion lymph node dissection for patients with micrometastatic disease. New tests offer promise to reveal new information to further risk-stratify patients based on gene expression profiling of tumors, but the literature surrounding the most well-known test is still nascent. The new insights into the pathogenesis and molecular basis for tumorigenesis have allowed a better understanding of who may be at risk for melanoma, in addition to groundbreaking new treatment strategies. As the burden of skin cancer increases across the United States and many other countries in northern and western Europe, the multidisciplinary scientific community rises to meet the challenge; new breakthroughs seem to be around every corner.

REFERENCES

1. American Cancer Society. Statistics for 2016. Available at: www.cancer.org/cancer/melanoma-skin-cancer.html. Accessed June 1, 2018.

2. American Academy of Dermatology. Melanoma fact sheet. Available at: www.aad.org/media/stats/conditions/melanoma-faqs. Accessed June 1, 2018.

3. Wagner JD, Gordon MS, Chuang TY, et al. Current therapy of cutaneous melanoma. Plast Reconstr Surg 2001;105:1774–99.

4. Sober AJ, Chuang TY, Duvic M, et al. Guidelines/outcomes committee. guidelines of care for primary cutaneous melanoma. J Am Acad Dermatol 2001; 45:579–86.

5. Tsao H. Update on familial cancer syndromes and the skin. J Am Acad Dermatol 2000;42:939–69.

6. Amaral T, Sinnberg T, Meier F, et al. The mitogen-activated protein kinase pathway in melanoma part I — Activation and primary resistance mechanisms to BRAF inhibition. Eur J Cancer 2017;73:85–92.

7. Gershenwald JE, Scolyer RA, Hess KR, et al. Melanoma staging: evidence-based changes in the American Joint Committee on Cancer eighth edition cancer staging manual. CA Cancer J Clin 2017; 67(6):472–92.

8. Skin Cancer Foundation. What is melanoma? Available at: www.skincancer.org/skin-cancer-information/melanoma. Accessed June 1, 2018.

9. Clinical practice guidelines: melanoma. National Comprehensive Cancer Network. Available at: www.nccn.org/professionals/physician_gls/PDF/melanoma.pdf. Accessed September 10, 2018.

10. Buzzell RA, Zitelli JA. Favorable prognostic factors in recurrent and metastatic melanoma. J Am Acad Dermatol 1996;34:798–803.

11. Ali-Salaam P, Ariyan S. Lymphatic mapping and sentinel lymph node biopsies. Clin Plast Surg 2000;27:421–9.

12. Murtha TD, Han G, Han D. Predictors for use of sentinel node biopsy and the association with improved survival in melanoma patients who have nodal staging. Ann Surg Oncol 2018;25(4):903–11.

13. Morton DL, Thompson JF, Cochran AJ, et al. Final trial report of sentinel-node biopsy versus nodal observation in melanoma. N Engl J Med 2014; 370(7):599–609.

14. Stiegel E, Xiong D, Ya J, et al. Prognostic value of sentinel lymph node biopsy according to Breslow thickness for cutaneous melanoma. J Am Acad Dermatol 2018;78(5):942–8.

15. Odom RB, James WD, Berger TG. Melanocytic nevi and neoplasms. In: James WD, Berger TG, Elston D, editors. Andrews' diseases of the skin. 9th edition. Philadelphia: WB Saunders; 2000. p. 881–9.

16. Novakovic B, Clark WH Jr, Fears TR, et al. Melanocytic nevi, dysplastic nevi, and malignant melanoma in children from melanoma-prone families. J Am Acad Dermatol 1995;33(4):631–6.

17. Greene M, Clark WH Jr, Tucker MA, et al. High risk of malignant melanoma in melanoma-prone families with dysplastic nevi. Ann Intern Med 1985;102:458–65.

18. Faries MB, Thompson JF, Cochran AJ, et al. Completion dissection or observation for sentinel-node metastasis in melanoma. N Engl J Med 2017; 376(23):2211–22.

19. Leiter U, Stadler R, Mauch C, et al. Complete lymph node dissection versus no dissection in patients with sentinel lymph node biopsy positive melanoma (DeCOG-SLT): a multicentre, randomised, phase 3 trial. Lancet 2016;17(6):757–67.

20. McMasters KM, Egger ME, Edwards MJ, et al. Final results of the Sunbelt Melanoma Trial: a multi-institutional prospective randomized phase III study evaluating the role of adjuvant high-dose interferon alfa-2b and completion lymph node dissection for patients staged by sentinel lymph node biopsy. J Clin Oncol 2016;34(10):1079–86.

21. Wong SL, Faries MB, Kennedy EB, et al. Sentinel lymph node biopsy and management of regional lymph nodes in melanoma: American Society of Clinical Oncology and Society of Surgical Oncology Clinical Practice Guideline Update. J Clin Oncol 2018;36(4):399–413.

22. Schuitevoerder D, Heath M, Cook RW, et al. Impact of gene expression profiling on decision-making in clinically node negative melanoma patients after surgical staging. J Drugs Dermatol 2018;17(2):196–9.

23. Gerami P, Cook RW, Wilkinson J, et al. Development of a prognostic genetic signature to predict the metastatic risk associated with cutaneous melanoma. Clin Cancer Res 2015;21(1):175–83.

24. Zager JS, Gastman BR, Leachman S, et al. Performance of a prognostic 31-gene expression profile in an independent cohort of 523 cutaneous melanoma patients. BMC Cancer 2018;18(1):130.

25. Ferris LK, Farberg AS, Middlebrook B, et al. Identification of high-risk cutaneous melanoma tumors is improved when combining the online American Joint Committee on Cancer Individualized Melanoma Patient Outcome Prediction Tool with a 31-gene expression profile-based classification. J Am Acad Dermatol 2017;76(5):818–25.

26. Shaikh WR, Dusza SW, Weinstock MA, et al. Melanoma thickness and survival trends in the United States, 1989 to 2009. J Natl Cancer Inst 2015; 108(1) [pii:djv294].

27. Ming ME. Commentary: the quest for an improved risk stratification tool for patients with melanoma. J Am Acad Dermatol 2017;76(5):826–8.

28. Gerami P, Cook RW, Russell MC, et al. Gene expression profiling for molecular staging of cutaneous melanoma in patients undergoing sentinel lymph node biopsy. J Am Acad Dermatol 2015;72(5):780–5.

29. Kosary CL, Altekruse SF, Ruhl J, et al. Clinical and prognostic factors for melanoma of the skin using SEER registries: collaborative stage data collection system, version 1 and version 2. Cancer 2014;120: 3807–14.

30. Greenhaw BN, Zitelli JA, Brodland DG. Estimation of prognosis in invasive cutaneous melanoma: an independent study of the accuracy of a gene expression profile test. Dermatol Surg 2018. [Epub ahead of print].

31. Hsueh EC, DeBloom JE, Lee J, et al. Interim analysis of survival in a prospective, multi-center registry cohort of cutaneous melanoma tested with a prognostic 31-gene expression profile test. J Hematol Oncol 2017;10(1):152.

32. Berger AC, Davidson RS, Poitras JK, et al. Clinical impact of a 31-gene expression profile test for cutaneous melanoma in 156 prospectively and consecutively tested patients. Curr Med Res Opin 2016; 32(9):1599–604.

33. Farberg AS, Glazer AM, White R, et al. Impact of a 31-gene expression profiling test for cutaneous melanoma on dermatologists' clinical management decisions. J Drugs Dermatol 2017;16(5):428–31.

34. Svoboda RM, Glazer AM, Farberg AS, et al. Factors affecting dermatologists' use of a 31-gene expression profiling test as an adjunct for predicting metastatic risk in cutaneous melanoma. J Drugs Dermatol 2018;17(5):544–7.

35. Olszanski AJ. Current and future roles of targeted therapy and immunotherapy in advanced melanoma. J Manag Care Spec Pharm 2014;20(4): 346–56.

36. Chapman PB, Hauschild A, Robert C, et al. Improved survival with vemurafenib in melanoma with BRAF V600E mutation. N Engl J Med 2011; 364(26):2507–16.

37. Hauschild A, Grob JJ, Demidov LV, et al. Dabrafenib in BRAF-mutated metastatic melanoma: a multicentre, open-label, phase 3 randomised controlled trial. Lancet 2012;380(9839):358–65.

38. Lugowska I, Koseła-Paterczyk H, Kozak K, et al. Trametinib: a MEK inhibitor for management of metastatic melanoma. Onco Targets Ther 2015;8:2251–9.

39. Ribas A, Gonzalez R, Pavlick A, et al. Combination of vemurafenib and cobimetinib in patients with advanced BRAF(V600)-mutated melanoma: a phase 1b study. Lancet Oncol 2014;15(9):954–65.

40. Long GV, Hauschild A, Santinami M, et al. Adjuvant dabrafenib plus trametinib in stage III BRAF-mutated melanoma. N Engl J Med 2017;377(19): 1813–23.

41. Wyman K, Atkins MB, Prieto V, et al. Multicenter phase II trial of high-dose imatinib mesylate in metastatic melanoma: significant toxicity with no clinical efficacy. Cancer 2006;106(9):2005–11.

42. Ugurel S, Hildenbrand R, Zimpfer A, et al. Lack of clinical efficacy of imatinib in metastatic melanoma. Br J Cancer 2005;92(8):1398–405.

43. Couzin-Frankel J. Breakthrough of the year 2013: cancer immunotherapy. Science 2013;342(6165): 1432–3.

44. Robert C, Thomas L, Bondarenko I, et al. Ipilimumab plus dacarbazine for previously untreated metastatic melanoma. N Engl J Med 2011;364(26):2517–26.

45. Maio M, Grob JJ, Aamdal S, et al. Five-year survival rates for treatment-naive patients with advanced melanoma who received ipilimumab plus dacarbazine in a phase III trial. J Clin Oncol 2015;33(10): 1191–6.

46. Hamid O, Puzanov I, Dummer R, et al. Final analysis of a randomised trial comparing pembrolizumab versus investigator-choice chemotherapy for ipilimumab-refractory advanced melanoma. Eur J Cancer 2017;86:37–45.

47. Schachter J, Ribas A, Long GV, et al. Pembrolizumab versus ipilimumab for advanced melanoma: final overall survival results of a multicentre, randomised, open-label phase 3 study (KEYNOTE-006). Lancet 2017;390(105):1853–62.

48. Robert C, Long GV, Brady B, et al. Nivolumab in previously untreated melanoma without BRAF mutation. N Engl J Med 2015;372(4):320–30.

49. Weber JS, D'Angelo SP, Minor D, et al. Nivolumab versus chemotherapy in patients with advanced melanoma who progressed after anti-CTLA-4 treatment (CheckMate 037): a randomised, controlled, open-label, phase 3 trial. Lancet Oncol 2015;16(4): 375–84.

50. Larkin J, Chiarion-Sileni V, Gonzalez R, et al. Combined nivolumab and ipilimumab or monotherapy in untreated melanoma. N Engl J Med 2015;373(1): 23–34.

Skin Cancer and Immunosuppression

Lindsey Collins, MD*, Andrew Quinn, MD, Thomas Stasko, MD

KEYWORDS

- Nonmelanoma skin cancer • Melanoma • Immunosuppression • Organ transplant recipients
- Mohs micrographic surgery • Squamous cell carcinoma • Chemoprevention
- Human papillomavirus

KEY POINTS

- Although survival rates of patients in immunosuppressed states, such as HIV, chronic lymphocytic leukemia, and post-transplant, are improving, the incidence of skin cancer in these populations continues to increase.
- Risk factors for skin cancers in immunosuppressed patients include those seen in the general population as well as others related to the degree of immunosuppression.
- Preventive strategies play an important role in immunosuppressed patients given their increased frequency and rapid development of new premalignant and malignant skin lesions.
- Integrated multidisciplinary care between the dermatology, dermatologic surgery, medical oncology, radiation oncology, and transplant teams is pivotal when caring for immunosuppressed patients with cutaneous malignancies.
- Evidence-driven guidelines regarding the preventative and therapeutic strategies for skin cancers in immunosuppressed patients are critical and should be sought by both clinicians and researchers.

INTRODUCTION

Immunosuppressed patients are at markedly increased risk of developing cutaneous malignancies compared with the general population. Although immunosuppression can result from a variety of conditions, the most studied population with regard to cutaneous malignancies is the organ transplant recipient cohort. Management of these patients requires an integrated multidisciplinary approach with dermatology, dermatologic surgery, medical oncology, radiation oncology, and the transplant team. Although there have been advances in the diagnosis and treatment of skin cancer in this high-risk population, there remains a lack of evidence-based therapeutic and preventive strategies to guide management.

EPIDEMIOLOGY OF IMMUNOSUPPRESSION

Transplant

There are 120,000 transplants performed worldwide each year, with more than 350,000 solid organ transplant recipients (SOTRs) in the United States as of 2016.[1–8] SOTRs have long been recognized as having a significantly increased risk of skin cancers. With increasing post-transplantation survival in SOTRs, the incidence continues to steadily increase.[1,9] Increased number of immunosuppressive medications, increased doses, and increased duration of immunosuppression have all been linked with increased incidence.[1]

Greater than 50% of white SOTRs are affected by skin cancer. Diagnosis is typically 3 years to

Disclosure Statement: None of the authors has any relationship with a commercial company that has a direct financial interest in subject matter or materials discussed in the article or with a company making a competing product.
Department of Dermatology, The University of Oklahoma Health Sciences Center, 619 Northeast 13th Street, Oklahoma City, OK 73104, USA
* Corresponding author.
E-mail address: Lindsey-collins@ouhsc.edu

Dermatol Clin 37 (2019) 83–94
https://doi.org/10.1016/j.det.2018.07.009

8 years after transplantation, with more than 90% of tumors being basal cell carcinoma (BCC) or squamous cell carcinoma (SCC). Many SOTRs are diagnosed with multiple tumors and these tumors tend to be more aggressive than those seen in the general population.[1,9] SCC, the most common type of skin cancer in SOTRs, has a 65-fold to 250-fold increased incidence over the general population, whereas BCC, the second most common type, has an incidence 10 times that of the general population (**Table 1**).[10] This situation is in contrast with the general population where BCC is diagnosed more frequently than SCC.[9]

Melanoma has a 2-fold to 5-fold increased incidence in SOTRs compared with the general population, with recent evidence showing a continual increase in incidence since 2000.[11,12] This increased risk is higher in African American SOTRs, with a 17-fold increased incidence over their immunocompetent peers.[1,13] In the pediatric SOTR population, the relative proportion of melanomas among skin cancers is higher than in adult recipients (12% vs 5% of all skin cancers, respectively).[14,15]

Other less common types of skin cancers that are diagnosed more frequently in SOTRs include Merkel cell carcinoma (MCC) and Kaposi sarcoma (KS) both of which have a viral etiopathogenesis. MCC has an incidence of 5 times to 50 times that seen in the general population whereas the risk of KS is increased 80-fold to 500-fold.[1,9]

Consistent with the general population, the risk of all skin cancers is much higher in white SOTRs versus nonwhite SOTRs, with the incidence of SCC in the white SOTR population 14 times that of the nonwhite SOTR population.[16] In contrast to the overall risk of skin cancer, the risk of skin cancer of the genital area is much higher in nonwhite SOTRs.[16]

In an American SOTR cohort of 120 patients in which a standardized genital skin examination had been adopted, 111 patients (92.5%) denied having genital lesions, but 53 (42.5%) were found to have lesions on examination. Of these, there were 7 malignant lesions in 6 patients, and all these patients were nonwhite.[16] This cohort highlights the importance of a special focus on malignancy screening of the genitalia in nonwhite SOTRs.

Chronic Lymphocytic Leukemia

Chronic lymphocytic leukemia (CLL), the most common leukemia of adults in the United States, has been associated with an increased risk of skin cancer.[17–19] These patients have an 8-fold increased risk of nonmelanoma skin cancer (NMSC) as well as a 2-fold to 4-fold increased incidence of melanoma.[17,19] These tumors also tend to be more aggressive, with NMSC demonstrating a higher rate of recurrence after Mohs surgery compared with the general population and a mortality rate in patients diagnosed with melanoma that is 2.5-times higher than the general population.[17,18,20]

HIV

The HIV-infected population has a risk of developing BCC and SCC that is increased 2-fold and 5-fold, respectively, of that of the general population.[21,22] The risk of NMSC, especially SCC, increases further in patients with poorly controlled HIV, who are subsequently more immunosuppressed (ie, CD4 <200 cells/mL and/or HIV viral load of $\geq$10,000 copies/mL).[9,21,23] The risk of BCC is increased only in the subset of HIV-infected patients who endorse the men who have sex with men (MSM) route of infection. It has been hypothesized that this may be due to a possible increased level of UV exposure that the MSM subset has over the overall HIV-infected population.[21]

Another important skin cancer in HIV is KS, which is considered an AIDS-defining illness.[24] With the introduction of antiretroviral therapy, the incidence of KS has decreased significantly, but it remains a common diagnosis in HIV-infected patients with a prevalence of 6%.[24,25]

Table 1
Relative risk associated with cutaneous malignancies in immunosuppressed patients

	Basal Cell Carcinoma	Squamous Cell Carcinoma	Melanoma	Merkel Cell Carcinoma	Kaposi Sarcoma
Transplant	10	65–250	2–5	5–50	80–500
CLL	8*	8*	2–4	—	—
HIV	2	5	1	2–10	100,000

* The combined relative risk for basal cell carcinoma and squamous cell carcinoma is 8.
   Data from Refs.[1,9,10,12,17,21,42,81]

Iatrogenic Immunosuppression for Autoimmune and Autoinflammatory Disease

There are currently many different biologic agents used in the treatment of psoriasis as well as psoriatic arthritis, rheumatoid arthritis, inflammatory bowel disease, and other autoinflammatory and autoimmune diseases. These include tumor necrosis factor inhibitors (TNFi) and inhibitors of the interleukin 17 pathway. Given the effect that these medications have on the immune system, a theoretically increased risk of skin cancer has been considered in creating psoriasis treatment guidelines.

Studies on psoriasis, rheumatoid arthritis, and inflammatory bowel disease patients have suggested an increased risk of NMSC, especially SCC, in patients exposed to TNFi.[26,27] Unlike NMSC, the risk of melanoma does not seem increased in patients exposed to TNFi.[27] More studies are needed to fully examine the risk of TNFi and other biologics on skin cancer.

RISK FACTORS FOR SKIN CANCERS IN IMMUNOSUPPRESSED PATIENTS
Nonmelanoma Skin Cancer

Independent risk factors for SCC in SOTRs include cumulative UV light exposure, history of NMSC prior to transplant, lower Fitzpatrick skin types, male gender, and age greater than 50 at time of transplantation.[1,2] Different types of organ transplants are also associated with higher risk of NMSC, with heart transplants carrying the highest risk followed by lung transplants. Kidney and liver transplant recipients have a lower risk, with most cohorts indicating that kidney transplant recipients have a higher risk than those receiving a liver.[1]

Risk of NMSC also increases with higher doses, longer duration, and increased numbers of immunosuppressive drugs, resulting in higher levels of immunosuppression. This increased immunosuppression helps explain, in part, the difference in risk in different types of organ transplants because heart and lung transplants require higher levels of immunosuppression.[1]

In patients who have been diagnosed with skin cancer prior to transplantation, the incidence after transplantation is increased 2.92-fold over those with no pretransplantation malignancy.[1,28]

Melanoma

It is hypothesized that the increased risk of melanoma is due to the decreased ability of the host immune system to recognize tumors and the increased surveillance regimens that these patients undergo in looking for all types of skin cancer.[12] Risk factors for melanoma include age greater than 50 years or less than 18 years at time of transplant, white race, family history of melanoma, high levels of UV exposure, high numbers of nevi, and a pretransplant history of melanoma.[9,12,29] Melanoma in the transplant population has been shown to be more aggressive compared with the general population and, when matched for Breslow thickness and Clark level, has been associated with worse outcomes.[1,29,30]

Merkel Cell Carcinoma

MCC has been associated with the Merkel cell polyomavirus, which has been detected in up to 80% of healthy adults over 50 years of age. Despite these high levels of exposure, it remains a rare tumor in the general population.[31] Given its viral etiology, it is not surprising that the immunosuppressed population has a 5-fold to 50-fold increased risk, with approximately 1 in 10 MCCs diagnosed in immunosuppressed patients.[1,31] The average age of onset in SOTRs is 53 years compared with the average age of 74 to 76 in the immunocompetent population.[31] MCC is typically diagnosed approximately 7.5 years post-transplantation and has a predilection for chronically sun-damaged areas, such as the head, neck, and arms.[9] The prognosis of MCC in SOTRs is much worse, with a 1-year survival rate of 47% versus 89% seen in the general population.

Kaposi Sarcoma

KS, caused by human herpesvirus 8 (HHV-8), is considered an AIDS-defining illness, with a prevalence of 6% in a recent HIV-infected cohort.[1,24] The risk decreases with increasing CD4, which explains the decreasing prevalence since the introduction of antiretroviral therapy.[24,25] The risk also varies in different geographic areas with HHV-8 seropositivity of less than 5% in North America and more than 50% in parts of Africa.[9]

Seropositivity in SOTRs prior to transplantation carries a far higher risk of developing KS of 23% to 28% compared with the 0.7% risk seen in seronegative patients. KS typically appears 13 months after transplantation[9] (Fig. 1).

PREVENTION STRATEGIES OF SQUAMOUS CELL CARCINOMA IN THE IMMUNOSUPPRESSED

Preventative strategies play an important role in immunosuppressed patients given their increased frequency and rapidity of developing premalignant and malignant skin lesions. Sun protection is a modifiable risk factor for the development of

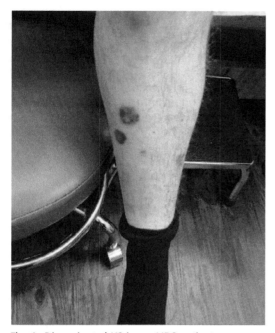

Fig. 1. Disseminated KS in an AIDS patient.

cutaneous malignancies and should be discussed with all immunosuppressed patients. Patients should receive extensive counseling regarding sun avoidance, the use of sunscreens, and the use of sun-protective clothing. Choosing the optimal treatment regimen for this population requires considering the extent of the disease, anatomic location involved, patient comorbidities, and patient preference. Actinic keratoses (AKs) have a risk of transforming into squamous cell carcinoma, thus providing a rationale for their aggressive treatment. Treatment strategies for AKs and actinically damaged skin include destruction techniques (cryotherapy, electrodessication and curettage, and carbon dioxide laser), shave removal, topical immunomodulators and chemotherapy agents, and photodynamic therapy.

Topical Chemoprevention

Topical 5-fluorouracil (5-FU) decreases the size and number of AKs and can be used in combination with alpha/beta hydroxy acids or topical tretinoin to increase penetration. In addition, the weekly application of 5-FU under occlusion with chemowraps is a well-tolerated therapeutic option for patients with widespread AKs of the extremities.[32]

A single report of acute renal failure in a patient treated with topical imiquimod for viral warts has limited its use in transplant patients[33]; however, there are many case reports and case series indicating that it is safe in transplant patients if applied over limited areas (60–100 cm^2).[34–36] There is a risk of cytokine release syndrome when imiquimod is applied over a large surface area, and more studies are needed to determine the associated risk in the immunosuppressed population.[37] Diclofenac 3% gel applied twice daily for 16 weeks has been shown effective in reducing AKs in organ transplant patients.[38]

Photodynamic Therapy

Photodynamic therapy with topical aminolevulinic acid is an effective treatment option for AKs as well as superficial NMSCs; however, there is a lack of data regarding long-term efficacy. A recent case series demonstrated that compared with imiquimod, photodynamic therapy obtained a higher rate of AK clearance at 3-month follow-up in organ transplant recipients. The study also showed shorter-lasting, but more intense, short-term skin reactions.[39]

Systemic Chemoprevention

In some cases, the rate and extent to which malignancies develop in immunosuppressed patients are too rapid for traditional surgical or field therapy. Medications for chemoprevention that have been studied in immunosuppressed patients include acitretin, nicotinamide, and capecitabine. These medications should be considered in patients who develop multiple squamous cell carcinomas per year (>5), aggressive squamous cell carcinomas, or accelerated development of squamous cell carcinomas.[40]

Acitretin has been used for the prevention and reduction of NMSCs. Acitretin should be started at a low dose of 10 mg per day and increased by 10-mg increments at 2-week to 4-week intervals to achieve the desired effect. The target dose is 20 mg/d to 25 mg/d.[41] After discontinuation, significant rebound in SCCs may occur.[42] A systematic review suggests that retinoids are safe for short-term use in organ transplant patients. Future studies are needed to establish long-term efficacy in this population.[43]

Nicotinamide, 500 mg twice daily, has been shown to decrease the incidence of AKs and NMSCs in immunocompetent patients; however, there is a lack of data in the immunosuppressed population.[44] In a recent phase II randomized controlled study, nicotinamide was associated with a statistically nonsignificant reduction of NMSCs and AKs in organ transplant patients.[45] Nicotinamide is available over the counter and is typically well tolerated with minimal side effects.

Low-dose oral capecitabine has been used for chemoprevention in patients who develop more than 2 cutaneous squamous cell carcinomas in 6 months; in those who continue to develop keratinocytic carcinomas despite treatments with oral retinoids, photodynamic therapy, or topical chemotherapies; or after optimization of immunosuppressive regimens.[46] Further studies are needed to establish the long-term efficacy of these chemoprevention modalities in immunosuppressed patients.

TREATMENT OF SQUAMOUS CELL CARCINOMA IN THE IMMUNOSUPPRESSED

Given that SCCs in organ transplant recipients seem more aggressive compared with immunocompetent patients, prompt, appropriate management of early disease is essential.[47] Aggressive surgical treatment is generally recommended, with Mohs micrographic surgery the optimum surgical approach for high-risk lesions and when tissue conservation is desired (Fig. 2). Although there is a lack of research on Mohs surgery in immunosuppressed patients, there is extensive data suggesting that it has the highest cure rate in immunocompetent patients. If a wide local excision is performed, the recommended surgical margins in the organ transplant population are between 3 mm and 10 mm; however, there is a lack of clinical data looking at residual and recurrent SCC using these margins in transplant patients.[48] The most effective treatment strategy for squamous cell carcinoma in situ is controversial in immunosuppressed patients secondary to the lack of long-term prospective studies comparing surgery versus other destructive modalities.[49]

Immunosuppressed patients are also at increased risk of developing eruptive keratoacanthomas compared with the general population.[50] Off-label treatment options, which have been reported in immunocompetent patients, include topical 5-FU, topical imiquimod, intralesional 5-FU, intralesional bleomycin, intralesional methotrexate, and topical 5-FU under zinc oxide chemowraps.[51–53]

Radiation therapy is reserved for patients with inoperable carcinomas, for those who cannot tolerate surgery, or for lesions that demonstrate extensive perineural involvement or incomplete resection.[49] There is a lack of existing data regarding the clinical benefit of sentinel lymph node biopsies in high-risk organ transplant recipients. There are currently no prospective studies indicating which patients are most likely to benefit from sentinel lymph node biopsies, making it difficult to assess the clinical benefit in these patients.

MODIFICATION IN IMMUNOSUPPRESSIVE REGIMENS

Immunosuppressive regimens in organ transplant patients are divided into induction, maintenance, and rejection therapy. Characteristics of the immunosuppressive regimen itself, including duration of therapy and type of medication, are important risk factors for the development of skin cancers. One of the most important adjuvant therapeutic strategies for managing immunosuppression-associated skin cancers is adjusting the immunosuppressive regimen. This requires collaboration with the entire transplant team. There are 3 main approaches to altering the immunosuppressive regimen in an effort to decrease the risk of skin cancers in transplant patients. The total immunosuppression level can be decreased, agents that seem to potentiate the carcinogenic process can be decreased, and/or the immunosuppressive agents that seem to inhibit the carcinogenic

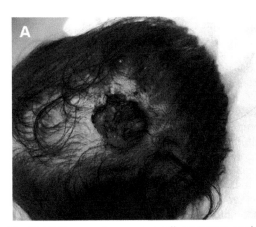 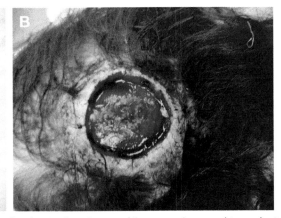

Fig. 2. (A) Recurrent squamous cell carcinoma on the scalp after Mohs micrographic surgery in a renal transplant patient. (B) Defect after 2 stages of Mohs micrographic surgery.

process can be added or increased.[54] The risk of graft rejection has to be strongly considered if the immunosuppressive regimen is altered.

The maintenance regimen often includes a calcineurin inhibitor (cyclosporin or tacrolimus), an antiproliferative agent (azathioprine or mycofenolate mofetil), and steroids, all which are known to increase the risk of cutaneous malignancies. Transplant teams are often more willing to be aggressive in decreasing immunosuppressive regimens in renal or liver transplant patients compared with cardiovascular or pulmonary transplant patients. Renal transplant patients have the option to return to dialysis if graft failure occurs. In addition, there is a history of tolerance to significant reductions in the immunosuppressive regimens in liver transplant patients and a greater ability of liver tissue to recover if rejection does occur.[55] The International Transplant Skin Cancer Collaborative (ITSCC) and Skin Care in Organ Transplant Patients Europe Reduction of Immunosuppression Task Force developed a consensus by a panel of experts regarding the level of tumor burden and risk of skin cancer warranting consideration of reduction of immunosuppression.[55] According to their recommendations, mild reduction of transplant-associated immunosuppression should be considered once multiple skin cancers per year develop or with individual high-risk skin cancers. Moderate reduction should be considered when patients experience greater than 25 skin cancers per year or for skin cancers with a 10% 3-year risk of mortality. Severe reduction should be considered only for life-threating skin cancers.[55]

Another option for transplant patients to decrease the incidence of cutaneous malignancies is to add a mammalian target of rapamycin (mTOR) inhibitor, a serine-threonine kinase that has an important regulatory function in cell growth and proliferation. By blocking this enzyme, mTOR inhibitors exhibit immunosuppressive effects via inhibition of B-cell and T cell proliferation. The medications in this class have both immunosuppressive effects and also the ability to partially reverse the oncogenic effects of other immunosuppressive agents.[54,56–58] The most studied medication in this class with regard to the effects on skin cancer is sirolimus; however, everolimus has also been shown to decrease the development of new skin cancers in transplant patients.[59–61] A majority of studies evaluating the effect of the addition of sirolimus to the immunosuppressive regimen have demonstrated a reduced incidence of skin cancer in renal organ transplant patients.[62,63] There are fewer data on the use of sirolimus for the prevention of skin cancer in nonrenal organ transplant patients. A recent 9-year retrospective mixed-organ cohort of organ transplant recipients demonstrates that patients taking sirolimus after developing post-transplant cancer had a lower risk of developing subsequent skin cancer, with no increased risk for overall mortality.[64] Further studies are needed to define the optimal conversion regimens and dosing in transplant patients and the effect of mTOR inhibitors initiated prior to the development of the first skin cancer. In addition, further studies are needed to determine the impact of sirolimus in patients who develop melanoma after transplant.

The specific immunosuppressive agent used may play an important role in the risk of developing skin cancers. Mycophenolate mofetil may mildly inhibit skin cancer development[54,65,66] compared with azathioprine. Conversion from azathioprine to mycophenolate mofetil should be considered in organ transplant recipients with multiple skin cancers.

SQUAMOUS CELL CARCINOMA STAGING IN IMMUNOSUPPRESSED PATIENTS

The American Joint Committee on Cancer (AJCC) issued the 8th edition of staging guidelines (AJCC8) in September 2016. The updated guidelines encompass tumors located on the head and neck only and have expanded the criteria for upstaging to stage T3. A recent retrospective cohort study comparing the AJCC 7th edition of staging guidelines (AJCC7) and AJCC8 tumor classification for head and neck squamous cell carcinoma demonstrated improved homogeneity and monotonicity in the AJCC8 staging system.[67] The prognostic accuracy of the 8th edition AJCC staging system has not yet been substantiated in the immunosuppressed population. A recent comparison of the AJCC7 and Brigham and Women's Hospital (BWH) cutaneous squamous cell carcinoma staging in immunosuppressed patients demonstrates that BWH staging criteria better risk stratifies cutaneous squamous cell carcinomas in immunosuppressed patients for risk of nodal metastasis and risk of local recurrence.[68] In the study, the majority of poor outcomes from SCC in the immunosuppressed patients occurred in low T stages.[68] There are no such studies comparing the AJCC7 or BWH staging system with the new AJCC8 staging system in immunosuppressed versus immunocompetent patients. Additional studies are needed to quantify the increased risk of poor outcomes for the same T-stage SCCs in immunocompetent versus immunocompromised patients and better risk stratification of low T-stage SCCs in immunosuppressed patients is needed. Immune status is not currently included as part of the staging criteria; however, given the higher risk of poor outcomes associated with immunosuppression, this should be considered in future staging systems. Early detection and definitive treatment is pertinent of even the low-stage SCC in the immunosuppressed cohort (Table 2).

MANAGEMENT OF MELANOMA IN IMMUNOSUPPRESSED PATIENTS

The management of localized melanoma in immunosuppressed patients parallels that of the immunocompetent population, with patients undergoing wide local excision with margins based on the Breslow thickness.[69] Sentinel lymph node testing should be discussed for patients with T1b melanoma according to the National Comprehensive Cancer Network 2018 treatment guidelines (<0.8 mm thick with ulceration and 0.8–1.0 mm thick without ulceration). Decision to defer sentinel lymph node biopsy may be based on comorbidities, patient preference, or other factors; however, data obtained from the biopsy may be beneficial in determining those who may benefit from reduction in the immunosuppressive regimen and/or other adjuvant treatment.

Although there have recently been significant advances in the treatment of patients with metastatic melanoma leading to improved survival rates, immunosuppressed patients were excluded from the pivotal immunotherapy studies. Given the lack of data on the use of immune checkpoint inhibitors in the immunosuppressed population, guiding care in these patients is difficult. The use of immune checkpoint inhibitors in SOTRs is controversial due to the risk of graft rejection, which has been documented.[70,71] Renal transplant patients may be better candidates for these medications given the possibility of returning to dialysis if rejection does occur. A recent case report described the first organ transplant patient with melanoma who received ipilimumab followed by nivolumab without experiencing a kidney allograft rejection.[72] Case reports have demonstrated that CTLA-4 inhibitors have a lower risk of allograft rejection than PD-1 inhibitors. PD-1 inhibitors mostly result in acute allograft rejection.[73] In mouse models, anti–CTLA-4 increased lethal graft versus host disease if given early after allogeneic stem cell transplant, but the effect on graft versus host disease was diminished if given late after marrow engraftment.[74] Late blockade of CTLA-4, once tolerance has been established, has been

Table 2
Comparison of squamous cell carcinoma staging systems

American Joint Committee on Cancer 7th Edition[a]		American Joint Committee on Cancer 8th Edition		Brigham and Women's Hospital[b]	
T Stage	Risk factors	T Stage	Risk factors (head and neck only)	T Stage	Risk factors
T1	Tumor ≤2 cm with <2 high-risk features	T1	Tumor diameter <2 cm	T1	No high-risk features
T2	Tumor >2 cm or tumor of any size with ≥2 high-risk factors	T2	Tumor diameter ≥2 cm and <4 cm in greatest dimension	T2a T2b	1 high-risk feature 2–3 high-risk features
T3	Tumor with invasion of maxilla, mandible, orbit, or temporal bone	T3	Tumor diameter ≥4 cm, or minor bone erosion, or perineural invasion or deep invasion	T3	≥4 high-risk features
T4	Tumor with invasion of skeleton or perineural invasion of skull base	T4	Tumor with gross cortical bone/marrow invasion	T4	Not applicable

[a] AJCC7 high-risk features: depth (>2 mm thickness; Clark level ≥IV), perineural invasion, location (primary site ear or nonglabrous lip), and differentiation (poorly differentiated or undifferentiated).
[b] BWH high-risk factors: tumor diameter ≥2 cm, invasion beyond subcutaneous fat, poorly differentiated, and perineural invasion.
Data from Karia PS, Morgan FC, Califano JA, et al. Comparison of tumor classifications for cutaneous squamous cell carcinoma of the head and neck in the 7th vs 8th edition of the AJCC cancer staging manual. JAMA Dermatol 2018;154(2):175–81; and Gonzalez JL, Cunningham K, Silverman R, et al. Comparison of the American Joint Committee on Cancer Seventh Edition and Brigham and Women's Hospital Cutaneous Squamous Cell Carcinoma Tumor Staging in Immunosuppressed Patients. Dermatol Surg 2017;43(6):784–91.

associated with graft survival.[75] Graft rejection has also been reported with immunostimulatory therapies, such as interferon.[76]

There are emerging data of promising combination therapies with mTOR, BRAF/MEK, and BTK/ITK inhibitors in transplant patients.[73] Prospective studies are needed to establish the best treatment regimen for transplant patients with advanced melanoma to optimize the antitumor response and minimize the risk of allograft rejection.

ITSCC has made evidence-based recommendations regarding the wait time before undergoing transplantation in patients with a prior history of a cutaneous malignancy, including melanoma (**Table 3**).[77] Although patients with distant metastatic disease are not eligible for transplantation in most circumstances, they may be considered as candidates following a wait time of 10 years to 15 years. According to the ITSCC

recommendations, the routine use of sentinel lymph node biopsy should be strongly considered in transplant candidates with melanoma less than 1.00 mm, because a negative sentinel lymph node biopsy may justify curtailing transplantation wait times on a case-by-case basis.

ROLE OF PATIENT EDUCATION AND HIGH RISK SPECIALTY CLINICS

Preventative dermatologic management is pivotal in the care of immunosuppressed patients. There should be integrated multidisciplinary care with dermatology, dermatologic surgery, medical oncology, radiation oncology, and the transplant team. Transplant patients who use sunscreen regularly have been found to have a decreased incidence of a second NMSCs after the diagnosis of the first.[78] The initial evaluation of a new transplant patient should include a detailed risk assessment to provide an index for the likelihood of developing subsequent skin cancers. This includes a detailed transplant history, skin cancer history, and full-body skin examination and lymph node examination. It is well documented that organ transplant recipients have insufficient knowledge regarding the importance of sun protection in addition to inadequate sun-protective behavior,[79] further indicating the need for more effective educational interventions and counseling for these patients. Patients should also be counseled regarding monthly self-skin examinations. Rigorous sun protection and early detection are key to the preventative management in these patients.

The frequency of skin cancer screenings depends on many factors, including patient risk factors, type of transplant, age at time of transplant, and type of immunosuppression regimen. Definitive guidelines have not yet been established regarding the recommended frequency of skin examinations in immunosuppressed patients. Expert consensus guidelines recommend a full-body skin examination every 12 months for organ transplant patients with no skin cancer history, every 6 months for patients with AKs or 1 keratinocytic carcinoma, every 3 months for those with multiple keratinocytic carcinomas or high-risk cutaneous squamous cell carcinoma, and every 1 month to 3 months for metastatic cutaneous squamous cell carcinoma.[49]

DISCUSSION/FUTURE TRENDS

Given the plethora of skin cancer complications secondary to immunosuppression, ongoing research and collaboration between clinicians and researchers are essential to better understand

Table 3
Recommended wait times pretransplant with a diagnosis of melanoma and squamous cell carcinoma

Skin Malignancy	Wait Time Before Transplantation After Treatment
Malignant melanoma	
In situ melanoma	No wait necessary, follow-up post -transplant 3 mo
Stage Ia melanoma	2 y
Stage Ib/IIa	2–5 y
Stage IIb/IIc	5 y
Any stage III or IV	Not eligible for transplantation
Cutaneous squamous cell carcinoma	
Low risk	No delay necessary
High risk SCC without perineural invasion	2 y
High-risk SCC with perineural invasion or ≥2 risk factors	2–3 y
High-risk with local nodal metastatic disease	5 y
Distant metastasis	No eligible for transplantation

Adapted from Zwald F, Leitenberger J, Zeitouni N, et al. Recommendations for solid organ transplantation for transplant candidates with a pretransplant diagnosis of cutaneous squamous cell carcinoma, merkel cell carcinoma and melanoma: a consensus opinion from the international transplant skin cancer collaborative (ITSCC). Am J Transplant 2016;16(2):140; with permission.

the disease pathogenesis and best management strategies for these patients. There now are formal consensus guidelines created by dermatologists and transplant physicians and endorsed by the ITSCC and the International Society of Heart and Lung Transplantation to help guide decision making with regard to immunosuppressed patients. Evidence-driven guidelines regarding the preventative and therapeutic strategies for skin cancers in immunosuppressed patients, however, are still needed.

Novel approaches to photoprotection are currently being investigated in organ transplant recipients. T4 endonuclease V, an enzyme involved in the repair of DNA damage after exposure to UV radiation, has been formulated as a lotion, and the safety and efficacy are currently being investigated in preventing keratinocytic carcinomas in organ transplant recipients.[49] In addition, afamelanotide, a more potent and longer-acting chemical analog of alpha-melanocyte-stimulating hormone, has been formulated as a subcutaneous pellet, and its efficacy in reducing AKs and cutaneous squamous cell carcinoma is being investigated in organ transplant patients.[49]

The role of the human papillomavirus (HPV) vaccination in the prevention of cutaneous squamous cell carcinoma is another topic of interest in the immunosuppressed population. β-HPV DNA is frequently associated with cutaneous squamous cell carcinomas in immunosuppressed patients. Currently, novel vaccines that offer cross-reactivity against β-HPV types are being developed and may hold promise in prevention of cutaneous squamous cell carcinoma.[80]

The development of skin cancer in immunosuppressed patients is a major clinical challenge and should be of continuous concern for dermatologists, transplant physicians, and patients.

REFERENCES

1. Howard MD, Su JC, Chong AH. Skin cancer following solid organ transplantation: a review of risk factors and models of care. Am J Clin Dermatol 2018;19(4):585–97.
2. Gogia R, Binstock M, Hirose R, et al. Fitzpatrick skin phototype is an independent predictor of squamous cell carcinoma risk after solid organ transplantation. J Am Acad Dermatol 2013;68(4):585–91.
3. Colvin M, Smith JM, Hadley N, et al. OPTN/SRTR 2016 annual data report: heart. Am J Transplant 2018;18(Suppl 1):291–362.
4. Hart A, Smith JM, Skeans MA, et al. OPTN/SRTR 2016 annual data report: kidney. Am J Transplant 2018;18(Suppl 1):18–113.
5. Smith JM, Weaver T, Skeans MA, et al. OPTN/SRTR 2016 annual data report: intestine. Am J Transplant 2018;18(Suppl 1):254–90.
6. Kandaswamy R, Stock PG, Gustafson SK, et al. OPTN/SRTR 2016 annual data report: pancreas. Am J Transplant 2018;18(Suppl 1):114–71.
7. Kim WR, Lake JR, Smith JM, et al. OPTN/SRTR 2016 annual data report: liver. Am J Transplant 2018; 18(Suppl 1):172–253.
8. Valapour M, Lehr CJ, Skeans MA, et al. OPTN/SRTR 2016 annual data report: lung. Am J Transplant 2018;18(Suppl 1):363–433.
9. Euvrard S, Kanitakis J, Claudy A. Skin cancers after organ transplantation. N Engl J Med 2003;348(17): 1681–91.
10. Wieland U, Kreuter A. Merkel cell polyomavirus infection and Merkel cell carcinoma in HIV-positive individuals. Curr Opin Oncol 2011;23(5):488–93.
11. Fattouh K, Ducroux E, Decullier E, et al. Increasing incidence of melanoma after solid organ transplantation: a retrospective epidemiological study. Transpl Int 2017;30(11):1172–80.
12. Robbins HA, Clarke CA, Arron ST, et al. Melanoma risk and survival among organ transplant recipients. J Invest Dermatol 2015;135(11):2657–65.
13. Hollenbeak CS, Todd MM, Billingsley EM, et al. Increased incidence of melanoma in renal transplantation recipients. Cancer 2005;104(9):1962–7.
14. Euvrard S, Kanitakis J, Cochat P, et al. Skin cancers following pediatric organ transplantation. Dermatol Surg 2004;30(4 Pt 2):616–21.
15. Penn I. Malignant melanoma in organ allograft recipients. Transplantation 1996;61(2):274–8.
16. Nadhan KS, Larijani M, Abbott J, et al. Prevalence and types of genital lesions in organ transplant recipients. JAMA Dermatol 2018;154(3):323–9.
17. Velez NF, Karia PS, Vartanov AR, et al. Association of advanced leukemic stage and skin cancer tumor stage with poor skin cancer outcomes in patients with chronic lymphocytic leukemia. JAMA Dermatol 2014;150(3):280–7.
18. Famenini S, Martires KJ, Zhou H, et al. Melanoma in patients with chronic lymphocytic leukemia and non-Hodgkin lymphoma. J Am Acad Dermatol 2015; 72(1):78–84.
19. Brewer JD, Shanafelt TD, Call TG, et al. Increased incidence of malignant melanoma and other rare cutaneous cancers in the setting of chronic lymphocytic leukemia. Int J Dermatol 2015;54(8): e287–93.
20. Mehrany K, Weenig RH, Pittelkow MR, et al. High recurrence rates of squamous cell carcinoma after Mohs' surgery in patients with chronic lymphocytic leukemia. Dermatol Surg 2005;31(1):38–42 [discussion: 42].
21. Omland SH, Ahlstrom MG, Gerstoft J, et al. Risk of skin cancer in HIV-infected patients: a Danish

nationwide cohort study. J Am Acad Dermatol 2018 [pii:S0190-9622(18)30475-4].

22. Silverberg MJ, Leyden W, Warton EM, et al. HIV infection status, immunodeficiency, and the incidence of non-melanoma skin cancer. J Natl Cancer Inst 2013;105(5):350–60.

23. Asgari MM, Ray GT, Quesenberry CP Jr, et al. Association of multiple primary skin cancers with human immunodeficiency virus infection, CD4 count, and viral load. JAMA Dermatol 2017;153(9):892–6.

24. Yarchoan R, Uldrick TS. HIV-associated cancers and related diseases. N Engl J Med 2018;378(11): 1029–41.

25. Gallafent JH, Buskin SE, De Turk PB, et al. Profile of patients with Kaposi's sarcoma in the era of highly active antiretroviral therapy. J Clin Oncol 2005; 23(6):1253–60.

26. Peleva E, Exton LS, Kelley K, et al. Risk of cancer in patients with psoriasis on biological therapies: a systematic review. Br J Dermatol 2018;178(1):103–13.

27. Chen Y, Friedman M, Liu G, et al. Do tumor necrosis factor inhibitors increase cancer risk in patients with chronic immune-mediated inflammatory disorders? Cytokine 2018;101:78–88.

28. Kang W, Sampaio MS, Huang E, et al. Association of pretransplant skin cancer with posttransplant malignancy, graft failure and death in kidney transplant recipients. Transplantation 2017;101(6):1303–9.

29. Puza CJ, Cardones AR, Mosca PJ. Examining the incidence and presentation of melanoma in the cardiothoracic transplant population. JAMA Dermatol 2018;154(5):589–91.

30. Vajdic CM, Chong AH, Kelly PJ, et al. Survival after cutaneous melanoma in kidney transplant recipients: a population-based matched cohort study. Am J Transplant 2014;14(6):1368–75.

31. Ma JE, Brewer JD. Merkel cell carcinoma in immunosuppressed patients. Cancers (Basel) 2014;6(3): 1328–50.

32. Peuvrel L, Saint-Jean M, Quereux G, et al. 5-fluorouracil chemowraps for the treatment of multiple actinic keratoses. Eur J Dermatol 2017;27(6): 635–40.

33. Santos-Juanes J, Esteve A, Mas-Vidal A, et al. Acute renal failure caused by imiquimod 5% cream in a renal transplant patient: review of the literature on side effects of imiquimod. Dermatology 2011; 222(2):109–12.

34. Das G, Tan B, Nicholls K. Safety and efficacy of a novel short occlusive regimen of imiquimod for selected non-melanotic skin lesions in renal transplant patients. Intern Med J 2016;46(3):352–5.

35. Brown VL, Atkins CL, Ghali L, et al. Safety and efficacy of 5% imiquimod cream for the treatment of skin dysplasia in high-risk renal transplant recipients: randomized, double-blind, placebo-controlled trial. Arch Dermatol 2005;141(8):985–93.

36. Ulrich C, Busch JO, Meyer T, et al. Successful treatment of multiple actinic keratoses in organ transplant patients with topical 5% imiquimod: a report of six cases. Br J Dermatol 2006;155(2):451–4.

37. Trakatelli M, Katsanos G, Ulrich C, et al. Efforts to counteract locally the effects of systemic immunosuppression: a review on the use of imiquimod, a topical immunostimulator in organ transplant recipients. Int J Immunopathol Pharmacol 2010;23(2):387–96.

38. Ulrich C, Johannsen A, Rowert-Huber J, et al. Results of a randomized, placebo-controlled safety and efficacy study of topical diclofenac 3% gel in organ transplant patients with multiple actinic keratoses. Eur J Dermatol 2010;20(4):482–8.

39. Togsverd-Bo K, Halldin C, Sandberg C, et al. Photodynamic therapy is more effective than imiquimod for actinic keratosis in organ transplant recipients: a randomized intraindividual controlled trial. Br J Dermatol 2018;178(4):903–9.

40. Otley CC, Stasko T, Tope WD, et al. Chemoprevention of nonmelanoma skin cancer with systemic retinoids: practical dosing and management of adverse effects. Dermatol Surg 2006;32(4):562–8.

41. Zwald FO, Brown M. Skin cancer in solid organ transplant recipients: advances in therapy and management: part II. Management of skin cancer in solid organ transplant recipients. J Am Acad Dermatol 2011;65(2):263–79 [quiz: 280].

42. Harwood CA, Leedham-Green M, Leigh IM, et al. Low-dose retinoids in the prevention of cutaneous squamous cell carcinomas in organ transplant recipients: a 16-year retrospective study. Arch Dermatol 2005;141(4):456–64.

43. Chen K, Craig JC, Shumack S. Oral retinoids for the prevention of skin cancers in solid organ transplant recipients: a systematic review of randomized controlled trials. Br J Dermatol 2005;152(3):518–23.

44. Yiasemides E, Sivapirabu G, Halliday GM, et al. Oral nicotinamide protects against ultraviolet radiation-induced immunosuppression in humans. Carcinogenesis 2009;30(1):101–5.

45. Chen AC, Martin AJ, Dalziell RA, et al. A phase II randomized controlled trial of nicotinamide for skin cancer chemoprevention in renal transplant recipients. Br J Dermatol 2016;175(5):1073–5.

46. Endrizzi B, Ahmed RL, Ray T, et al. Capecitabine to reduce nonmelanoma skin carcinoma burden in solid organ transplant recipients. Dermatol Surg 2013;39(4):634–45.

47. Martinez JC, Otley CC, Stasko T, et al. Defining the clinical course of metastatic skin cancer in organ transplant recipients: a multicenter collaborative study. Arch Dermatol 2003;139(3):301–6.

48. Stasko T, Brown MD, Carucci JA, et al. Guidelines for the management of squamous cell carcinoma in organ transplant recipients. Dermatol Surg 2004; 30(4 Pt 2):642–50.

49. Blomberg M, He SY, Harwood C, et al. Research gaps in the management and prevention of cutaneous squamous cell carcinoma in organ transplant recipients. Br J Dermatol 2017;177(5):1225–33.

50. Kwiek B, Schwartz RA. Keratoacanthoma (KA): an update and review. J Am Acad Dermatol 2016; 74(6):1220–33.

51. Ribero S, Balagna E, Sportoletti Baduel E, et al. Efficacy of electrochemotherapy for eruptive legs keratoacanthomas. Dermatol Ther 2016;29(5):345–8.

52. Metterle L, Nelson C, Patel N. Intralesional 5-fluorouracil (FU) as a treatment for nonmelanoma skin cancer (NMSC): a review. J Am Acad Dermatol 2016;74(3):552–7.

53. Tallon B, Turnbull N. 5% fluorouracil chemowraps in the management of widespread lower leg solar keratoses and squamous cell carcinoma. Australas J Dermatol 2013;54(4):313–6.

54. Ritchie SA, Patel MJ, Miller SJ. Therapeutic options to decrease actinic keratosis and squamous cell carcinoma incidence and progression in solid organ transplant recipients: a practical approach. Dermatol Surg 2012;38(10):1604–21.

55. Otley CC, Berg D, Ulrich C, et al. Reduction of immunosuppression for transplant-associated skin cancer: expert consensus survey. Br J Dermatol 2006; 154(3):395–400.

56. Euvrard S, Morelon E, Rostaing L, et al. Sirolimus and secondary skin-cancer prevention in kidney transplantation. N Engl J Med 2012;367(4):329–39.

57. Kauffman HM, Cherikh WS, Cheng Y, et al. Maintenance immunosuppression with target-of-rapamycin inhibitors is associated with a reduced incidence of de novo malignancies. Transplantation 2005;80(7): 883–9.

58. Geissler EK. Skin cancer in solid organ transplant recipients: are mTOR inhibitors a game changer? Transplant Res 2015;4:1.

59. Euvrard S, Boissonnat P, Roussoulieres A, et al. Effect of everolimus on skin cancers in calcineurin inhibitor-treated heart transplant recipients. Transpl Int 2010;23(8):855–7.

60. Alter M, Satzger I, Schrem H, et al. Non-melanoma skin cancer is reduced after switch of immunosuppression to mTOR-inhibitors in organ transplant recipients. J Dtsch Dermatol Ges 2014;12(6):480–8.

61. Caroti L, Zanazzi M, Paudice N, et al. Conversion from calcineurin inhibitors to everolimus with low-dose cyclosporine in renal transplant recipients with squamous cell carcinoma of the skin. Transplant Proc 2012;44(7):1926–7.

62. Smith A, Niu W, Desai A. The effect of conversion from a calcineurin inhibitor to sirolimus on skin cancer reduction in post-renal transplantation patients. Cureus 2017;9(8):e1564.

63. Knoll GA, Kokolo MB, Mallick R, et al. Effect of sirolimus on malignancy and survival after kidney transplantation: systematic review and meta-analysis of individual patient data. BMJ 2014;349: g6679.

64. Karia PS, Azzi JR, Heher EC, et al. Association of sirolimus use with risk for skin cancer in a mixed-organ cohort of solid-organ transplant recipients with a history of cancer. JAMA Dermatol 2016; 152(5):533–40.

65. Coghill AE, Johnson LG, Berg D, et al. Immunosuppressive medications and squamous cell skin carcinoma: nested case-control study within the skin cancer after organ transplant (SCOT) cohort. Am J Transplant 2016;16(2):565–73.

66. Einollahi B, Nemati E, Lessan-Pezeshki M, et al. Skin cancer after renal transplantation: results of a multicenter study in Iran. Ann Transplant 2010;15(3): 44–50.

67. Karia PS, Morgan FC, Califano JA, et al. Comparison of tumor classifications for cutaneous squamous cell carcinoma of the head and neck in the 7th vs 8th edition of the AJCC Cancer Staging Manual. JAMA Dermatol 2018;154(2):175–81.

68. Gonzalez JL, Cunningham K, Silverman R, et al. Comparison of the American Joint Committee on Cancer Seventh Edition and Brigham and Women's Hospital Cutaneous Squamous Cell Carcinoma Tumor Staging in Immunosuppressed Patients. Dermatol Surg 2017;43(6):784–91.

69. Zwald FO, Christenson LJ, Billingsley EM, et al. Melanoma in solid organ transplant recipients. Am J Transplant 2010;10(5):1297–304.

70. Ranganath HA, Panella TJ. Administration of ipilimumab to a liver transplant recipient with unresectable metastatic melanoma. J Immunother 2015;38(5): 211.

71. Spain L, Higgins R, Gopalakrishnan K, et al. Acute renal allograft rejection after immune checkpoint inhibitor therapy for metastatic melanoma. Ann Oncol 2016;27(6):1135–7.

72. Herz S, Hofer T, Papapanagiotou M, et al. Checkpoint inhibitors in chronic kidney failure and an organ transplant recipient. Eur J Cancer 2016;67: 66–72.

73. Chae YK, Galvez C, Anker JF, et al. Cancer immunotherapy in a neglected population: the current use and future of T-cell-mediated checkpoint inhibitors in organ transplant patients. Cancer Treat Rev 2018;63:116–21.

74. Blazar BR, Taylor PA, Panoskaltsis-Mortari A, et al. Opposing roles of CD28:B7 and CTLA-4:B7 pathways in regulating in vivo alloresponses in murine recipients of MHC disparate T cells. J Immunol 1999; 162(11):6368–77.

75. Cecchini M, Sznol M, Seropian S. Immune therapy of metastatic melanoma developing after allogeneic bone marrow transplant. J Immunother Cancer 2015;3:10.

76. Greenberg JN, Zwald FO. Management of skin cancer in solid-organ transplant recipients: a multidisciplinary approach. Dermatol Clin 2011;29(2):231–41, ix.

77. Zwald F, Leitenberger J, Zeitouni N, et al. Recommendations for solid organ transplantation for transplant candidates with a pretransplant diagnosis of cutaneous squamous cell carcinoma, merkel cell carcinoma and melanoma: a consensus opinion from the international transplant skin cancer collaborative (ITSCC). Am J Transplant 2016;16(2):407–13.

78. Terhorst D, Drecoll U, Stockfleth E, et al. Organ transplant recipients and skin cancer: assessment of risk factors with focus on sun exposure. Br J Dermatol 2009;161(Suppl 3):85–9.

79. Robinson JK, Rigel DS. Sun protection attitudes and behaviors of solid-organ transplant recipients. Dermatol Surg 2004;30(4 Pt 2):610–5.

80. Kwak K, Jiang R, Wang JW, et al. Impact of inhibitors and L2 antibodies upon the infectivity of diverse alpha and beta human papillomavirus types. PLoS One 2014;9(5):e97232.

81. McGarvey ME, Tulpule A, Cai J. Emerging treatments for epidemic (AIDS-related) Kaposi's sarcoma. Curr Opin Oncol 1998;10(5):413–21.

Going Viral 2019
Zika, Chikungunya, and Dengue

Jose Dario Martinez, MD[a],*, Jesus Alberto Cardenas-de la Garza, MD[b],
Adrian Cuellar-Barboza, MD[b]

KEYWORDS

- Arbovirus • *Aedes aegypti* • Travel-related illness • Zika • Microcephaly • Chikungunya • Dengue

KEY POINTS

- Arbovirus infections, especially Zika, chikungunya, and dengue, have become international public health concerns. These 3 maladies share the same vector.
- Dermatologic manifestations, predominantly maculopapular rash, are frequently observed in travelers to endemic countries, particularly in Asia and South America.
- Zika is characterized by pruritic rash, low-grade fever, and arthralgia. Guillain-Barré syndrome and congenital nervous system malformations are severe complications.
- Chikungunya's hallmark is an intense arthralgia/arthritis that may become chronic; dermatologic findings include rash and facial melanosis.
- Dengue is the most frequent arbovirus infection worldwide and is potentially life threatening.

OVERVIEW

Chikungunya virus and Zika virus infections are emerging diseases in the Americas, and dengue virus continues to be the most prevalent arthropod-borne virus in the world. Medical problems in returned travelers are fever, acute diarrhea, and skin lesions that include rash. These arbovirus diseases may spread by endemic transmission or as travel-related infections, have rapidly expanded their geographic distribution, and, because of the world globalization, threaten millions of people. Furthermore, arbovirus infections (arthropod-borne virus) are increasingly important causes of neurologic disease in the Americas.

ZIKA VIRUS
Introduction

Zika is an enveloped, single-stranded RNA flavivirus primarily transmitted to humans through *Aedes*

spp mosquitoes. This rapidly emerging arbovirus infection has reached global scale since its arrival to the Americas in 2015. More than 2 billion people live in tropical and subtropical regions of the world with suitable environments for disease dissemination.[1] The association of Zika with Guillain-Barré syndrome (GBS) and congenital birth defects highlights the need for awareness of potential cases and how to diagnose, prevent, and treat this disease.[2]

History

Zika was first isolated in April 1947 from the blood of a rhesus macaque monkey in the Zika forest of Uganda. Nine months later, Zika was isolated from *Aedes africanus* mosquitoes collected from the same forest. In 1952, the first human cases of Zika were documented in patients from Uganda and Tanzania.[3] Until the early twenty-first century, only approximately a dozen mild cases of Zika

Disclosure Statement: The authors have nothing to disclose.
[a] Department of Internal Medicine, University Hospital "Dr. José E. González", UANL, Mitras Centro, Avenida Gonzalitos y Madero S/N, Monterrey 64460, Mexico; [b] Department of Dermatology, University Hospital "Dr. José E. González", Universidad Autónoma de Nuevo León, Mitras Centro, Avenida Gonzalitos y Madero S/N, Monterrey 64460, Mexico
* Corresponding author.
E-mail address: jdariomtz@yahoo.com.mx

derm.theclinics.com

fever were reported in countries confined to an equatorial zone across Africa and Asia.[4] In 2007, however, the first large outbreak outside mainland Africa and Asia occurred in Micronesia.[5] In 2013, a second major epidemic arose in French Polynesia, affecting approximately 270,000 people. Zika arrived to the Americas in 2015, presumably transmitted by mosquitoes or travelers, with numerous cases of human infections in Brazil.[3,6] Since then, the virus spread rapidly by mosquito-borne transmission and has been reported in 48 countries in the Americas.[4] In January 2016, the first case of Zika infection in the United States was diagnosed in Harris County, Texas.[7]

Microbiology and Transmission

Zika is a 50-nm, enveloped, and icosahedral particle belonging to the *Flavivirus* genus (from the Flaviviridae family) of single positive-strand RNA viruses.[8]

Other pathogens included in this family are DNV, West Nile virus, and yellow fever virus. There are 2 recognized lineages of Zika, African and Asian.[9] The neurologic complications, such as GBS and microcephaly, have only been linked to the Asian lineage; this strain was suspected to cause the Brazilian epidemic of Zika. To date, the influence of Zika genetic variation on its pathogenicity is not well understood.[10]

Zika is mainly transmitted through the bite of infected *A aegypti* mosquitos; these are morphologically characterized by a bright lyre-shaped dorsal pattern with white bands on its legs.[4] Both *A aegypti* and *A albopictus* are present in the southern and southeastern half of the United States, with peak abundance of them from June to October each year.[11]

Other member of the *Aedes* genus, as well as a variety of other mosquito species, such as *Culex quinquefasciatus*, have been linked to the infection.[12,13] There are 2 distinct transmission cycles: a sylvatic cycle, affecting nonhuman primates, and an urban cycle involved in the transmission between humans and urban mosquitos in towns. Mosquitoes that can spread Zika usually live in places below 2000 m. The probabilities of getting Zika fever from mosquitoes living above that altitude are very low.[14,15] Zika can also be passed from mother to child during pregnancy or spread through sexual contact, organ transplantation, or blood transfusion.[10] Zika has been detected in breast milk, yet no Zika transmission has been reported through breastfeeding.[16] The small potential of Zika transmission during breastfeeding may be outweighed by its known benefits.[17] The versatility of transmission modes in Zika infection

increases the difficulty of developing effective control strategies.

Epidemiology

The global risk of Zika spread remains high, particularly in the Americas region, although some countries have reported a decline in cases. The World Health Organization (WHO) reports more than 80 countries from Asia, Pacific Islands, America, and Africa with evidence of current vector-borne Zika transmission.[18]

Excluding pregnancy-derived Zika infection, in the United States more than 5500 symptomatic Zika fever vector-borne cases have been reported. Approximately 94% of those cases were from returned travelers.[19] Relevant countries from America with ongoing outbreaks are Venezuela, Brazil, Mexico, Colombia, El Salvador, Martinique, and Panama. Previously 2 regions from te continental United States (Brownsville, Texas, and Miami-Dade County, Florida) reported local mosquito-borne transmission. As of March 2018, the US Centers for Disease Control and Prevention (CDC) has lifted this warning.[19] The United States has a registry reporting more than 2400 pregnant women with laboratory evidence of possible Zika from 2015 to 2018, with more than 100 birth defects and approximately 10 pregnancy losses.[20]

Clinical Manifestations

Zika has an incubation period ranging from 3 days to 12 days. Only approximately 20% of individuals experience symptoms during Zika infection. These include mild fever (37.8°C–38.5°C), arthralgias predominantly of small joints in hands and feet, headache, myalgia, nonpurulent conjunctivitis in half of patients, and retroorbital pain[21–23] (**Fig. 1**). Dermatologists must be aware that approximately

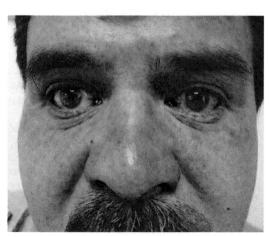

Fig. 1. Red eye in a patient with Zika.

90% of symptomatic Zika fever patients develop a rash.[23] Skin manifestations appear within 1 day to 4 days of symptoms (ie, fever and arthralgias), usually last 6 days (2–14 days), and are characterized by a pruritic maculopapular rash predominantly localized to the trunk and extremities, followed by the face[24,25] (**Fig. 2**). Palms and soles may be affected and the palate may show petechiae.[23,26] Fever is not a hallmark sign of this infection. The maculopapular rash is more sensitive for detecting Zika.[24,27] Rare clinical manifestations reported include thrombocytopenia, facial edema, uveitis, transient hearing impairment, myocarditis, pericarditis, and hematospermia.[25]

Clinical manifestations of children and infants with postnatal acute vector-borne ZKIV infection are similar to findings in adult patients. Previous reports have not found growth impairment in children with postnatal acquired disease.[28]

Zika infection has been related to neurologic complications, such as GBS, encephalitis, transverse myelitis, encephalomyelitis, meningoencephalitis, chronic inflammatory demyelinating polyneuropathy, brain ischemia, and neuropsychiatric symptoms.[29–32]

A case-control study of the Zika outbreak in French Polynesia reported 42 GBS cases related to Zika; 88% of these patients had Zika infection symptoms and the median interval between viral syndrome and onset of neurologic symptoms was 6 days; 38% of this population required intensive care management; and 29% needed respiratory care, but all of them survived. The incidence of GBS was estimated to be 2.4 cases per 10,000 Zika infections.[33]

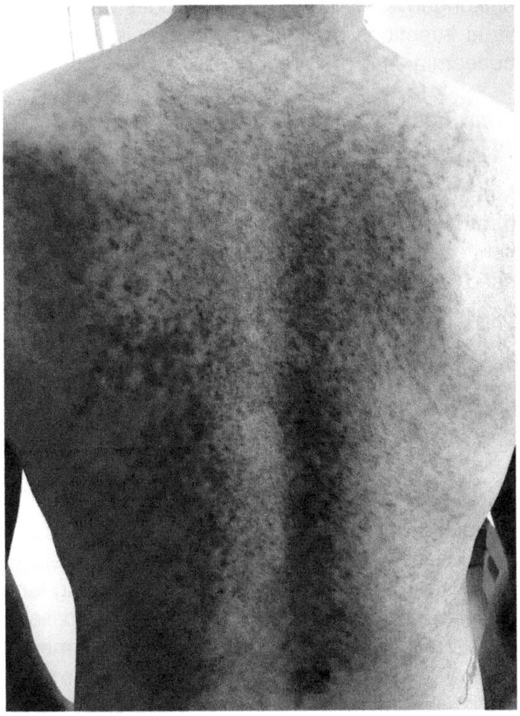

Vertical transmission during pregnancy of Zika virus may lead to severe teratogenic effects on the fetal nervous system. Pregnant women who had adverse congenital outcomes were 4 times more likely to have a history of a rash during pregnancy.[34] Women have the highest risk of acquiring congenital Zika syndrome if infected in the first trimester. Clinical manifestations of congenital Zika infection include microcephaly, hearing loss, ocular abnormalities, arthrogryposis, neuromotor abnormalities, seizures, and small-for-gestational age.[35,36] A prospective study from the French Territories in the Americas followed more than 500 symptomatic pregnant women with confirmed Zika infection; severe neurologic birth defects consistent with congenital Zika syndrome were diagnosed in 6.9% of first-trimester infections, 1.2% of second-trimester infections, and 0.9% of third-trimester infections.[37] Sperm count may drop between day 7 and day 30 after Zika infection but they generally normalize by day 120.[38] **Table 1** summarizes differences between Zika, chikungunya, and dengue.

Diagnosis

Zika infection may be established using real-time reverse transcription–polymerase chain reaction (RT-PCR) for RNA in serum, urine, or whole blood. This test has a sensibility and specificity of approximately 100%. In the United States; the patient should be given the CDC form (50.34) to take to a commercial laboratory for the specimen to be sent to the CDC.[39] For patients within 2 weeks of symptom onset, RT-PCR of serum and urine for detection of Zika RNA should be performed. Serum Zika RNA may be detectable within 2 days of symptom onset and up to 7 days afterward. Paired specimen analysis (urine and serum) is supported because evidence suggests urine RNA may appear later than it does in serum.[40,41] A positive result confirms the diagnosis; however, a negative result does not exclude Zika infection, especially several weeks after symptoms start and further serologic testing must be done. Diagnosis can be established with serology of immunoglobulin M (IgM) antibodies using IgM antibody capture (MAC)-ELISA with the confirmatory plaque reduction neutralization test (PRNT).[9,40] A PRNT titer greater than 10 for Zika with a Dengue PRNT titer less than 10 confirms Zika infection.

Fig. 2. Pruritic maculopapular trunk rash in Zika.

Table 1
Features between dengue, chikungunya, and Zika infections

Feature	Dengue	Chikungunya	Zika
Vector	*Aedes* spp	*Aedes* spp	*Aedes* spp
Geographic area	Worldwide	Worldwide	Worldwide
Incubation	5–8 d	1–12 d	3–12 d
Asymptomatic	60%–80%	<30%	>80%
Fever ≥39°C	+++	+++	++
Rash	+	++	+++
Arthralgia/myalgia	+/++	+++/+	++/+
Arthritis	−	+++	++
Bleeding	++	−	−
Lymphocytopenia	++	+++	+
Neutropenia	+++	++	+
Thrombocytopenia	+++	−	−
Chronic arthritis	−	+	−
GBS	+/−	+/−	+
Shock	+	−	−
Sexual transmission	−	−	+
Blood transfusion transmission	+/−	+/−	+
Microcephaly	−	−	+
Vaccine	Yes (not Food and Drug Administration approved)	No	No
Prevention	DEET	DEET	DEET

There is a potential risk for false-negative results during the serologic window because IgM antibodies are detectable 1 week to 2 weeks after symptom onset and remain detectable for several weeks.[40,42] IgG antibodies have little diagnostic value. All serologic methods can cross-react with other flaviviruses, in particular dengue.[9] A single laboratory RT-PCR test is available to evaluate for presence of Zika, Chikungunya, or Dengue infection. Because laboratory tests take longer than 24 hours to obtain confirmatory results, patients must be advised to avoid mosquito bites to potentially prevent local transmission.[24]

Pregnant women with possible exposure to Zika and symptoms must be tested promptly; paired analysis of both nucleic acid testing and IgM serology is recommended. Testing is not routinely advised but should be considered for pregnant and asymptomatic women with history of temporal exposure to Zika.[40] All pregnant women with laboratory tests suggestive or diagnostic of Zika infection should undergo prenatal ultrasonography 4 weeks after the suspected exposure. A nucleic acid Zika test in amniotic fluid is diagnostic of fetal viral exposure but not predictive of outcome, so tailored decisions by the clinician and the patient must be done.[43]

Differential diagnosis is similar between Zika, chikungunya, and dengue. It includes other arbovirus infections, malaria, leptospirosis, meningococcemia, and drug reactions.

Treatment

There is no specific medication for Zika infection. Management consists of rest and symptomatic treatment. Advising adequate fluid intake may prevent dehydration, and acetaminophen can be used as supportive therapy for fever and pain. Aspirin and other nonsteroidal anti-inflammatory drugs (NSAIDS) should be avoided until other viral infections have been ruled out.[24] Mosquito bed nets should be used in hospitalized patients to avoid further transmission.

Prevention

Population in areas with risk of transmission should take personal preventive measures to avoid arthropod bites; these include wearing long sleeves and long pants, using insect repellent, and staying indoors as feasible. Environmental control measures are aimed to eliminate mosquito-breeding sites. Individuals should prevent water from collecting in flowerpots, buckets, bottles, and jars.[44] Mosquito nets should be used in beds for prevention in endemic countries.

The CDC recommends the use of Environmental Protection Agency–registered insect repellents that have been confirmed as effective. They must contain 1 of the following elements: N,N-diethyl-meta-toluamide (DEET), para-menthane-3,8-diol, picaridin, oil of lemon eucalyptus, or IR3535. They must be applied on clothing, and in the skin. The CDC recommends waiting 6 months for men and 8 weeks for women before unprotected sex after symptom onset or last possible Zika exposure to prevent sexual transmission.[45]

Approximately 20 Zika vaccine candidates are being tested with different strategies: inactivated viruses, virus-like particles, recombinant viruses, and DNA vaccines. Three DNA vaccines that target prM/E proteins are on clinical trials. A phase 2 trial with a Zika wild-type DNA vaccine (VRC 5288) is currently ongoing.[46]

CHIKUNGUNYA FEVER
Introduction

Chikungunya fever is a re-emergent disease caused by the Chikungunya, an RNA alphavirus belonging to the Togaviridae family. It is transmitted via mosquito bite usually by Aedes spp, in particular A albopictus and A aegypti. Previously confined to Africa and Asia, rapid spread of Chikungunya since 2004 has become a public health concern. Introduction in 2013 to Caribbean islands resulted in spread to more than 40 countries in North and South America.[47]

History

Chikungunya derives from the Makonde dialect, meaning "that which bends up," and referring to the arthropathy caused by the virus.[48] Chikungunya probably caused epidemics in the nineteenth century in the Caribbean and the United States and has caused periodic epidemics in Asia every 4 decades to 5 decades. The virus was first isolated in Tanzania in 1952 and occasional outbreaks were detected in the following decades in several African and Asian nations. It is yet unknown when Chikungunya first originated.[14]

In 2004, a new epidemic strain developed in Kenya and swiftly expanded the following year to several islands in the Indian Ocean, including the French Island of La Réunion.[49] Concurrently, from 2005 to 2007, millions of cases were reported in India. A albopictus transmission adaption, travel, and Chikungunya mutations probably contributed to the swift dissemination[47,50] In 2007, the first autochthonous European cases were reported in Italy.[51] In America, Chikungunya

was first confirmed on the Caribbean in the Saint Martin island. The disease quickly spread through the Americas and transmission has been reported in 45 American nations.[14] Although in many new affected countries, A albopictus was the main vector, in many American countries both A albopictus and A aegypti were responsible for disseminating the infection.

Microbiology and Transmission

Chikungunya is an enveloped, single-stranded, positive-sense RNA virus belonging to the genus Alphavirus and family Togaviridae.[47,51] Other arbovirus in the Alphavirus genus include the Eastern equine encephalitis virus and the Mayaro virus.[52] Four Chikungunya lineages have been identified: West African; Eastern, Central, and Southern African; Asian; and the more recently determined Indian Ocean lineage.[49,53] Mutations have rendered these lineages diverse in their species of Aedes mosquito transmission.

A aegypti (also known as yellow fever mosquito) is the most prevalent vector in tropical and subtropical climates. It is also responsible for other arbovirus transmitted infections like dengue, Zika, and yellow fever. It is widely distributed wordwide and is well adapted to urban and periurban settings.[54] Since 2006, A albopictus (also known as the Asian tiger mosquito) became a mayor transmission vector partially secondary to mutations rendering increased infectivity and smaller dissemination time in this specie.[52]

Both species lay their eggs on small water-filled containers. A aegypti usually bites in daylight (dawn and dusk), indoors or outdoors, takes multiple bloodmeals, and is more anthropophilic than A albopictus.[14] Humans represent the principal Chikungunya reservoirs during epidemics. During the enzootic cycle, nonhuman primates and other vertebrates are suspected to be the principal reservoirs.[50] Vertical transmission (mother-to-child) is also present and is associated with a high morbidity. Blood products in endemic areas should be screened for Chikungunya due to possible transmission.[48]

Epidemiology

Chikungunya transmission is now encountered on all 5 continents. Africa and Asia are the regions most affected. In 2016 in the Americas, more than 300,000 cases (with almost 150,000 laboratory confirmed) were recorded. The countries most affected were Brazil, Bolivia, and Colombia.[55] Continental United States had few locally transmitted cases in 2014 and 2015.[56] Data from 2017 revealed more than 100 chikungunya cases from 26 states of the United States, all from returning travelers. California, New York, and Texas were the states with the most cases.[57] Local transmission in Italy and France was reported in 2017.[58]

Clinical Manifestations

Chikungunya has an incubation period ranging from 1 day to 12 days (most often 3–7 days). Approximately 75% of cases are symptomatic. Manifestations start abruptly with fever, arthralgia/arthritis, myalgia, and headache. The polyarthritis is usually inflammatory and symmetri, and affects more frequently the hands, wrists, ankles, and knees. Axial and periarticular involvement may be present.[59] Articular symptoms are a hallmark of the disease and are usually more severe than in other common arboviruses. The most common dermatologic manifestation is a maculopapular rash involving the trunk and limbs that appears 2 days to 5 days after the fever starts (**Fig. 3**). It may be slightly pruritic or asymptomatic and can affect the palms and soles. Although classically described as sparing the face, some cases present with facial or nasal erythema.[60] The rash presence is variable among series ranging from 30% to 75% of cases.[48] Macular hyperpigmentation is the second most common dermatologic manifestations presenting as localized (nasal or centrofacial melasma–like) or

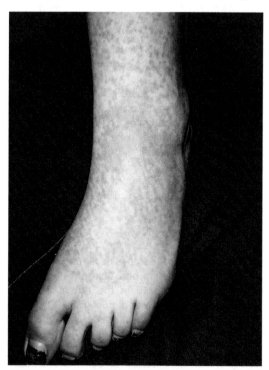

Fig. 3. Chikungunya fever transient rash.

disseminated pigmentation, which can have a freckled or confetti-like appearance. Nose pigmentation has been dubbed, *chik sign*, because it has not been described in other similar infections. Genital, oral, or intertriginous painful ulcers have been described. A vesiculobullous eruption in children is an infrequent chikungunya presentation, which poses a diagnostic challenge. Other dermatologic signs include purpura and melanonychia.[48,60,61]

Different from other arbovirus, chikungunya may present long-lasting, chronic articular manifestations that may persist for months to years. These symptoms, included under the term, *post-chikungunya chronic inflammatory rheumatism*, include arthritis, arthralgias, myalgia, and tenosynovitis, which resemble rheumatoid arthritis or psoriatic arthritis. Significant compromise of the quality of life and indirect economic loss is a major concern.[62,63] Congenital and perinatal transmission is associated with severe manifestations, including meningoencephalitis and long-term neurocognitive sequelae.[64] Risk factors for severe disease and complications include vertical transmission, older age, initial severe acute disease, and comorbidities. The mortality rate of chikungunya is very low and is usually secondary to complications of preexisting diseases or central nervous system involvement.

Diagnosis

The most useful tool for early Chikungunya diagnosis is real-time RT-PCR, which has excellent sensitivity and specificity. It can detect Chikungunya during the first week when serologic evaluation may be falsely negative. Serologic IgM assays become positive 2 days to 6 days after symptoms and persist elevated for 3 months to 6 months. Chikungunya IgG elevation is positive after the first week of symptoms and persist for years. Longitudinal evaluation for 4-fold IgG antibody titer increase is suggestive of chikungunya infection. Serologic assays may have cross-reactivity with other mosquito-borne infections.[39,48,50,65] Rash biopsy findings are unspecific (spongiosis, dermal edema, and perivascular lymphocytic infiltrate). Hyperpigmented lesions show pigment incontinence, basal layer hyperpigmentation, and melanophages.[48,60]

Treatment

There is currently no specific antiviral treatment or vaccine against Chikungunya. Treatment is supportive with rest, pain and fever control, and hydration. Fever should be managed with acetaminophen. Analgesics like NSAIDs are recommended for articular symptoms.[48,59,62,65] Comorbidities must be evaluated for exacerbations. Chronic articular symptoms require rheumatological evaluation. Therapy with methotrexate and antimalarials in post-chikungunya chronic inflammatory rheumatism has shown variable results.[59,62]

Prevention

Personal and environmental preventive measures to avoid arthropod bites are the same as discussed for Zika. No vaccine is currently approved for chikungunya. Currently, 18 Chikungunya vaccine candidates are under assessment. Two vaccines are in phase 2 trials.[46]

DENGUE
Introduction

Dengue is the most frequent mosquito-borne infection in the world.[66] It is potentially fatal and timely diagnosis and treatment is fundamental. It shares common vectors as other arbovirus. Coinfections carry higher morbidity. The etymology of the word dengue probably originated to the Swahili phrase, "Ka dinga pepo," which means a kind of sudden cramp-like seizure from an evil spirit. These words were then interconnected to the Spanish dengue and the English dandy, alluding to the fastidious and manneristic walks, respectively, associated with painful movement.[67]

History

Dengue (also known as dandy fever and breakbone fever) descriptions date back to the third century in China.[68] After the seventeenth century, the rising prevalence was concurrent with increasing maritime trade.[68,69] Several investigators have argued the possibility that several historical outbreaks of dengue fever were misclassified and correspond to Chikungunya.[70]

Epidemiology

Dengue is endemic is more than 125 countries, mostly subtropical and tropical regions.[71] Approximately half of the world population inhabits dengue endemic countries. Yearly incidence ranges 50 million to 100 million cases, with approximately 20,000 deaths attributed. Global burden is most dominant in Latin America and Asia.[72] Projections state that dengue incidence is likely to expand in the future.[71]

Microbiology and Transmission

Dengues include 4 serologic distinct RNA viruses that belong to the genus Flavivirus and family Flaviviridae. All 4 serotypes can cause the disease. Within each Dengue genotype, genetic variations can further classify them into genotypes with different virulence profiles. This variability hinders the production of vaccines protective to all dengue subtypes.[68,73] Infection with one serotype produces long-term (sometimes lifetime) immunity to that serotype but only short-term immunity to other ones. Second infection is an important risk factor for presenting severe disease.[66,73] The 4 serotypes have varying geographic distribution and some countries have endemic transmission of all. Antibody-dependent enhancement is a phenomenon that occurs when antibodies to other dengue serotypes produces non-neutralizing antibodies to other serotypes promoting viral replication and subsequently additional disease severity. This phenomenon raises concern that vaccines with limited efficacy to some serotypes may exacerbate infections with these serotypes.[66,73]

A aegypti is the most common vector. Geographic spread of A albopictus raises concern about its future role in dengue expansion in A aegypti nonendemic regions.[72]

Clinical Manifestations

Dengue has a diverse clinical presentation that ranges from mild disease to severe, life-threatening complications. Prediction of outcome is challenging. Only 20% of infected patients manifest clinical disease. Dengue has a short incubation period of 5 days to 8 days. The first phase of the infection (febrile phase) is characterized by sudden fever, retroorbital pain, and myalgia/arthralgia. Face, neck, or trunk flushing is the first dermatologic manifestation occurring in the first 24 hours to 48 hours (**Fig. 4**). Subsequently, a faint morbilliform rash (classically described as isles of white in a sea of red) that may be mildly pruritic is present in more than 50% of cases.

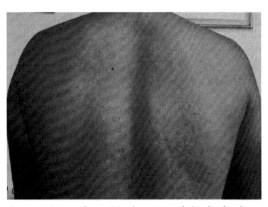

Fig. 4. Faint and pruritic dengue rash in the back.

Hemorrhagic manifestations may appear in this phase and include petechiae, ecchymosis, and mucosal bleeding. Leukopenia in this phase is suggestive of dengue infection.[74,75] The tourniquet test consists of inflating the blood pressure cuff for 5 minutes, intermediate of systolic and diastolic blood pressure. The appearance of more than 10 petechia in 1 cm^2 of skin is a specific sign of dengue.[76] Defervescence occurs 3 days to 7 days after symptom begin. Although most patients recover after this phase, some patients may develop symptoms secondary to capillary leakage (critical phase). This period lasts 1 days to 2 days. Leukopenia, thrombocytopenia, hematocrit elevation, ascites, and pleural effusion occur. Shock may develop with organ failure secondary to hypoperfusion. The recovery phase lasts 2 days to 3 days and is characterized by fluid reabsorption and white blood cell, hematocrit, and platelet normalization. The morbilliform rash can be present in this phase. Hypervolemia secondary to excessive intravenous fluid administration can lead to complications.[75]

The WHO simplified dengue classification into 3 categories—dengue without warning signs, dengue with warning signs, and severe dengue. Probable dengue is defined as a clinical scenario in a patient that lives or has traveled to a dengue endemic area and presents with fever and 2 of the following: nausea/vomiting, rash, leukopenia, positive tourniquet test, aches/pains, or any warning sign. Persistent vomiting, fluid accumulation, mucosal bleeding, lethargy/restlessness, hepatomegaly (>2 cm), and hematocrit increase with thrombocytopenia are considered warning signs. Severe dengue is considered in the presence of severe plasma leakage (shock and respiratory distress), severe bleeding, or organ failure.[75] Close monitorization of warning sign improves outcome.

Diagnosis

Clinical diagnosis alone is complicated and, whenever possible, laboratory evaluation must be performed. In primoinfection, serologic IgM assays become positive approximately 3 days to 5 day after the first symptoms. At day 3 to day 5, a positive test is found in half of the patients, progressing in day 10 to a 99% positivity. IgM titers decline and become undetectable after 2 months to 3 months. IgG antibodies become positive after the first week and can persist for life. In secondary infections, IgG titers rapidly rise early, whereas IgM persists low. IgM/IgG ratio lower than 1.2 or 1.4 implies secondary infection.[75] Other flavivirus infections can provoke cross-reactivity or false-

positive tests.[77] In endemic areas with other circulating flavivirus, other diagnostic methods are preferred.

Detection of NS1 antigen is available in several commercial assays. In primary infection, the test is positive during the first 9 days. In secondary infections, this period is shorter and antigen levels have been associated with severe disease.[77] The NS1 glycoprotein is not exclusive of Dengue and commercial kits may cross-react with other flavivirus like Zika. Assays that can identify between different dengue serotypes and other flavivirus are currently under development.[78] PCR is a sensitive and specific diagnostic method that can identify single or multiple dengue serotypes concomitantly. It is especially useful during the first 4 days to 5 days of infection.[66,77,78] Differential diagnosis is broad and includes other arboviral infections, influenza, mononucleosis, and rickettsial infections.

Treatment

No specific antiviral treatment is available. Treatment is supportive. Acetaminophen is recommended for pain and fever control. NSAIDs and aspirin should be avoided because of bleeding complications. Severe cases require inpatient care. Patients with signs of shock need ICU transferal. Tachycardia and hypoperfusion must be continuously evaluated as patient condition can swiftly deteriorate. Repeated complete blood cell counts are recommended. Careful fluid management is of paramount importance to avoid shock/overload. No specific treatment of bleeding complications is currently available and blood product transfusion is to be performed cautiously due to the possibility of pulmonary edema.[79]

Prevention

Prevention techniques common to other mosquito-borne diseases are recommended. A tetravalent vaccine of chimeric attenuated viruses has been approved.[80] High efficacy is reported in serotypes Dengue-3 and Dengue-4, moderate in Dengue-1, and low Dengue-2.[46,81] Recent follow-up has led to recognition of increased risk of severe dengue and hospitalizations in previously seronegative, vaccinated individuals. This may lead to a scarce benefit of this vaccine in low prevalence populations. Due to the increased risk of serious infection in previously seronegative population, and until further review, the WHO recommends this vaccine only in individuals with previous, confirmed dengue infection. Revised recommendations probably will be available soon.[80]

SUMMARY

These emerging arbovirus infections—Zika, chikungunya, and dengue—occur worldwide, and billions of people are at risk. For US residents, they are travel-related diseases, and prevention with appropriate clothing and insect repellents is basic. Counseling to travelers, especially for Zika, is important. Clinicians must be aware of clinical presentation as well for differential diagnosis with other maladies. Serology confirmation is essential. To date there are no Food and Drug Administration–approved vaccines, and management is supportive.

REFERENCES

1. Messina JP, Kraemer MU, Brady OJ, et al. Mapping global environmental suitability for Zika virus. Elife 2016;5:e15272.
2. Fauci AS, Morens DM. Zika virus in the Americas—yet another arbovirus threat. N Engl J Med 2016; 374:601–4.
3. Mlacker S, Shafa G, Aldahan AS, et al. Origin of the Zika virus revealed: a historical journey across the world. Int J Dermatol 2016;55: 1369–72.
4. Song B-H, Yun S-I, Woolley M, et al. Zika virus: history, epidemiology, transmission, and clinical presentation. J Neuroimmunol 2017;308:50–64.
5. Ioos S, Mallet H-P, Leparc Goffart I, et al. Current Zika virus epidemiology and recent epidemics. Med Mal Infect 2014;44:302–7.
6. Goorhuis A, von Eije KJ, Douma RA, et al. Zika virus and the risk of imported infection in returned travelers: implications for clinical care. Travel Med Infect Dis 2016;14:13–5.
7. McCarthy M. First US case of Zika virus infection is identified in Texas. BMJ 2016;352:i212.
8. Kostyuchenko VA, Lim EXY, Zhang S, et al. Structure of the thermally stable Zika virus. Nature 2016;533: 425–8.
9. Relich RF, Loeffelholz M. Zika virus. Clin Lab Med 2017;37:253–67.
10. Wang L, Valderramos SG, Wu A, et al. From mosquitos to humans: genetic evolution of Zika virus. Cell Host Microbe 2016;19:561–5.
11. Monaghan AJ, Morin CW, Steinhoff DF, et al. On the seasonal occurrence and abundance of the zika virus vector mosquito aedes aegypti in the contiguous United States. PLoS Curr 2016;8 [pii: ecurrents].
12. Guerbois M, Fernandez-Salas I, Azar SR, et al. Outbreak of Zika virus infection, Chiapas State, Mexico, 2015, and first confirmed transmission by aedes aegypti mosquitoes in the Americas. J Infect Dis 2016;214:1349–56.
13. Vasievich MP, Villarreal JDM, Tomecki KJ. Got the travel bug? a review of common infections, infestations, bites, and stings among returning travelers. Am J Clin Dermatol 2016;17:451–62.
14. Weaver SC, Barrett ADT. Transmission cycles, host range, evolution and emergence of arboviral disease. Nat Rev Microbiol 2004;2:789–801.
15. Center for Disease Control and Prevention. World Map of Areas with Risk of Zika. In: Travelers' Health. 2018. Available at: https://wwwnc.cdc.gov/travel/page/world-map-areas-with-zika. Accessed May 29, 2018.
16. Sotelo JR, Sotelo AB, Sotelo FJB, et al. Persistence of Zika Virus in Breast Milk after Infection in Late Stage of Pregnancy. Emerg Infect Dis 2017;23: 856–7.
17. The American College of Obstetricians and Gynecologists. Practice advisory interim guidance for care of obstetric patients during a Zika Virus outbreak. in: practice advisories. 2017. Available at: https://www.acog.org/Clinical-Guidance-and-Publications/Practice-Advisories/Practice-Advisory-Interim-Guidance-for-Care-of-Obstetric-Patients-During-a-Zika-Virus-Outbreak. Accessed May 29, 2018.
18. Center for Disease Control and Prevention. Zika travel information. In: Travelers' Health. 2018. Available at: https://wwwnc.cdc.gov/travel/page/zika-information. Accessed May 29, 2018.
19. Center for Disease Control and Prevention. Cumulative Zika Virus Disease Case Counts in the United States, 2015-2018. 2018. In: Zika Virus. Avaiable at: https://www.cdc.gov/zika/reporting/case-counts.html. Accessed May 29, 2018.
20. Center for Disease Control and Prevention. Pregnant women with any laboratory evidence of possible Zika virus infection, 2015-2018. In: Zika and pregnancy. 2018. Available at: https://www.cdc.gov/pregnancy/zika/data/pregwomen-uscases.html. Accessed May 29, 2018.
21. Yadav S, Rawal G, Baxi M. Zika virus: a pandemic in progress. J Transl Int Med 2016;4:42–5.
22. Basarab M, Bowman C, Aarons EJ, et al. Zika virus. BMJ 2016;352:i1049.
23. Derrington SM, Cellura AP, McDermott LE, et al. Mucocutaneous findings and course in an adult with Zika virus infection. JAMA Dermatol 2016;152: 691–3.
24. He A, Brasil P, Siqueira AM, et al. The emerging Zika virus threat: a guide for dermatologists. Am J Clin Dermatol 2017;18:231–6.
25. Pinto Junior VL, Luz K, Parreira R, et al. Zika virus: a review to clinicians. Acta Med Port 2015;28: 760–5.
26. Veletzky L, Knafl D, Schuster C, et al. Zika virus-induced itching rash in a returning traveller from Brazil. Int J Infect Dis 2017;54:13–4.

27. Brasil P, Calvet GA, Siqueira AM, et al. Zika virus outbreak in rio de janeiro, brazil: clinical characterization, epidemiological and virological aspects. PLoS Negl Trop Dis 2016;10:e0004636.

28. Li J, Chong CY, Tan NW, et al. Characteristics of Zika virus disease in children: clinical, hematological, and virological findings from an outbreak in Singapore. Clin Infect Dis 2017;64:1445–8.

29. da Silva IRF, Frontera JA, Bispo de Filippis AM, et al. Neurologic complications associated with the Zika virus in Brazilian adults. JAMA Neurol 2017;74:1190–8.

30. Mecharles S, Herrmann C, Poullain P, et al. Acute myelitis due to Zika virus infection. Lancet 2016;387:1481.

31. Carteaux G, Maquart M, Bedet A, et al. Zika virus associated with meningoencephalitis. N Engl J Med 2016;374:1595–6.

32. Zucker J, Neu N, Chiriboga CA, et al. Zika virus-associated cognitive impairment in adolescent, 2016. Emerg Infect Dis 2017;23:1047–8.

33. Cao-Lormeau VM, Blake A, Mons S, et al. Guillain-Barre Syndrome outbreak associated with Zika virus infection in French Polynesia: a case-control study. Lancet 2016;387:1531–9.

34. van den Worm L, Khumalo NP. Skin manifestations are common and associated with a higher prevalence of congenital abnormalities in Zika virus infection. Int J Dermatol 2017;56:1470–3.

35. Grossi-Soyster EN, LaBeaud AD. Clinical aspects of Zika virus. Curr Opin Pediatr 2017;29:102–6.

36. Brasil P, Pereira JPJ, Moreira ME, et al. Zika virus infection in pregnant women in Rio de Janeiro. N Engl J Med 2016;375:2321–34.

37. Hoen B, Schaub B, Funk AL, et al. Pregnancy outcomes after Zika infection in French territories in the Americas. N Engl J Med 2018;378:985–94.

38. Joguet G, Mansuy J-M, Matusali G, et al. Effect of acute Zika virus infection on sperm and virus clearance in body fluids: a prospective observational study. Lancet Infect Dis 2017;17:1200–8.

39. Korman AM, Alikhan A, Kaffenberger BH. Viral exanthems: an update on laboratory testing of the adult patient. J Am Acad Dermatol 2017;76:538–50.

40. Rabe IB, Staples JE, Villanueva J, et al. Interim guidance for interpretation of Zika virus antibody test results. MMWR Morb Mortal Wkly Rep 2016;65:543–6.

41. Campos R de M, Cirne-Santos C, Meira GLS, et al. Prolonged detection of Zika virus RNA in urine samples during the ongoing Zika virus epidemic in Brazil. J Clin Virol 2016;77:69–70.

42. Bingham AM, Cone M, Mock V, et al. Comparison of test results for Zika virus RNA in urine, serum, and saliva specimens from persons with travel-associated zika virus disease - Florida, 2016. MMWR Morb Mortal Wkly Rep 2016;65:475–8.

43. Adebanjo T, Godfred-Cato S, Viens L, et al. Update: interim guidance for the diagnosis, evaluation, and management of infants with possible congenital zika virus infection - United States, October 2017. MMWR Morb Mortal Wkly Rep 2017;66:1089–99.

44. LaRocque RL, Ryan ET. Personal actions to minimize mosquito-borne illnesses, including Zika virus. Ann Intern Med 2016;165:589–90.

45. Center for Disease Control and Prevention. Prevention and transmission. In: Zika virus. 2018. Available at: https://www.cdc.gov/zika/prevention/. Accessed May 29, 2018.

46. Silva JVJJ, Lopes TRR, Oliveira-Filho EF, et al. Current status, challenges and perspectives in the development of vaccines against yellow fever, dengue, Zika and chikungunya viruses. Acta Trop 2018;182:257–63.

47. Burt FJ, Chen W, Miner JJ, et al. Chikungunya virus: an update on the biology and pathogenesis of this emerging pathogen. Lancet Infect Dis 2017;17:e107–17.

48. Handler MZ, Handler NS, Stephany MP, et al. Chikungunya fever: an emerging viral infection threatening North America and Europe. Int J Dermatol 2017;56:e19–25.

49. Weaver SC, Forrester NL. Chikungunya: evolutionary history and recent epidemic spread. Antiviral Res 2015;120:32–9.

50. Mathew AJ, Ganapati A, Kabeerdoss J, et al. Chikungunya infection: a global public health menace. Curr Allergy Asthma Rep 2017;17:13.

51. Wahid B, Ali A, Rafique S, et al. Global expansion of chikungunya virus: mapping the 64-year history. Int J Infect Dis 2017;58:69–76.

52. Marcondes CB, Contigiani M, Gleiser RM. Emergent and reemergent arboviruses in South America and the Caribbean: why so many and why now? J Med Entomol 2017;54:509–32.

53. Lo Presti A, Cella E, Angeletti S, et al. Molecular epidemiology, evolution and phylogeny of Chikungunya virus: an updating review. Infect Genet Evol 2016;41:270–8.

54. Kraemer MUG, Sinka ME, Duda KA, et al. The global distribution of the arbovirus vectors Aedes aegypti and Ae. albopictus. Elife 2015;4:e08347.

55. World Health Organization. Chikungunya. In: WHO Fact sheets. 2017. Available at: http://www.who.int/en/news-room/fact-sheets/detail/chikungunya. Accessed May 29, 2018.

56. Staples J, Hills SL, Powers AM. Chikungunya. In: Brunette GW, editor. CDC yellow book 2018: health information for international travel. New York: Oxford University Press; 2017. p. 151–3.

57. Center for Disease Control and Prevention. 2017 provisional data for the United States. In: Chikungunya Virus. 2018. Available at: https://www.cdc.

gov/chikungunya/geo/united-states-2017.html. Accessed May 29, 2018.

58. World Health Organization. Chikungunya. In: Disease outbreaks news. 2018. Available at: http://www.who.int/csr/don/archive/disease/chikungunya/en/. Accessed May 29, 2018.

59. Vijayan V, Sukumaran S. Chikungunya virus disease: an emerging challenge for the rheumatologist. J Clin Rheumatol 2016;22:203–11.

60. Kumar R, Sharma MK, Jain SK, et al. Cutaneous manifestations of chikungunya fever: observations from an outbreak at a tertiary care hospital in Southeast Rajasthan, India. Indian Dermatol Online J 2017;8:336–42.

61. Singal A. Chikungunya and skin: current perspective. Indian Dermatol Online J 2017;8:307–9.

62. Sharma SK, Jain S. Chikungunya: a rheumatologist's perspective. Int J Rheum Dis 2018;21:584–601.

63. Rodriguez-Morales AJ, Cardona-Ospina JA, Fernanda Urbano-Garzon S, et al. Prevalence of post-chikungunya infection chronic inflammatory arthritis: a systematic review and meta-analysis. Arthritis Care Res (Hoboken) 2016;68:1849–58.

64. Torres JR, Falleiros-Arlant LH, Duenas L, et al. Congenital and perinatal complications of chikungunya fever: a Latin American experience. Int J Infect Dis 2016;51:85–8.

65. Kucharz EJ, Cebula-Byrska I. Chikungunya fever. Eur J Intern Med 2012;23:325–9.

66. Pang T, Mak TK, Gubler DJ. Prevention and control of dengue-the light at the end of the tunnel. Lancet Infect Dis 2017;17:e79–87.

67. Rigau-Perez JG. The early use of break-bone fever (Quebranta huesos, 1771) and dengue (1801) in Spanish. Am J Trop Med Hyg 1998;59:272–4.

68. Weaver SC, Vasilakis N. Molecular evolution of dengue viruses: contributions of phylogenetics to understanding the history and epidemiology of the preeminent arboviral disease. Infect Genet Evol 2009;9:523–40.

69. Holbrook MR. Historical perspectives on flavivirus research. Viruses 2017;9:97.

70. Kuno G. A re-examination of the history of etiologic confusion between dengue and chikungunya. PLoS Negl Trop Dis 2015;9:e0004101.

71. Murray NEA, Quam MB, Wilder-Smith A. Epidemiology of dengue: past, present and future prospects. Clin Epidemiol 2013;5:299–309.

72. World Health Organization. Global strategy for dengue prevention and control, 2012-2020. Geneve (Switzerland): WHO Press; 2012.

73. Thomas SJ, Endy TP. Current issues in dengue vaccination. Curr Opin Infect Dis 2013;26:429–34.

74. Thomas EA, John M, Kanish B. Mucocutaneous manifestations of Dengue fever. Indian J Dermatol 2010;55:79–85.

75. World Health Organization. Dengue: guidelines for diagnosis, treatment, prevention and control. Geneve (Switzerland): WHO Press; 2009.

76. Grande AJ, Reid H, Thomas E, et al. Tourniquet test for dengue diagnosis: systematic review and meta-analysis of diagnostic test accuracy. PLoS Negl Trop Dis 2016;10:e0004888.

77. Muller DA, Depelsenaire ACI, Young PR. Clinical and laboratory diagnosis of dengue virus infection. J Infect Dis 2017;215:S89–95.

78. Bosch I, de Puig H, Hiley M, et al. Rapid antigen tests for dengue virus serotypes and Zika virus in patient serum. Sci Transl Med 2017;9 [pii: eaan1589].

79. Lee TH, Lee LK, Lye DC, et al. Current management of severe dengue infection. Expert Rev Anti Infect Ther 2017;15:67–78.

80. World Health Organization. Updated questions and answers related to the dengue vaccine Dengvaxia® and its use. In: WHO immunization, vaccines and biologicals. 2018. Available at: http://www.who.int/immunization/diseases/dengue/revised_SAGE_recommendations_dengue_vaccines_apr2018/en/. Accessed May 29, 2018.

81. Villar L, Dayan GH, Arredondo-Garcia JL, et al. Efficacy of a tetravalent dengue vaccine in children in Latin America. N Engl J Med 2015;372:113–23.

Cosmeceuticals
What's Real, What's Not

Zoe Diana Draelos, MD

KEYWORDS

- Cosmeceuticals • Cleansers • Toners • Surfactants • Moisturizers • Peptides • Botanicals
- Skin lightening

KEY POINTS

- Cosmeceutical regimens incorporate cleansers and moisturizers as the backbone of the therapeutic regimen.
- Toners, cleansing scrubs, cleansing cloths, and mechanized devices all combine surfactant-based cleansing with exfoliation to improve skin smoothness and increase light reflection from the skin surface.
- Cleanser mildness may be evaluated using the collagen swelling test, pH rise test, or zein test.
- Skin-lightening cosmeceuticals are moving away from the use of hydroquinone and instead incorporating ingredients, such as liquiritin, isoliquertin, aloesin, arbutin, and vitamin C.
- Antiaging cosmeceutical moisturizers may use some of the newly developed peptides (carrier peptides, signal peptides, and neurotransmitter peptides) or topical vitamins to support their claims.

INTRODUCTION

The word, *cosmeceutical*, implies to the consumer a product purchased without prescription that profoundly affects skin appearance and functioning. From a regulatory standpoint, cosmeceuticals are simply cosmetics and nothing more. Consumers no longer wish to purchase products that scent and adorn the skin momentarily until removed. They are willing to pay a premium price for a cosmeceutical product that promises and delivers more skin benefits. The ability to charge a premium price has attracted the attention of manufacturers, dramatically increasing the cosmeceutical category offerings. This tremendous diversity in product availability provides meaningful products and products that are of minimal benefit, leading to the title of this article, promising to evaluate what is real and what is not.

COSMECEUTICAL CLEANSING TECHNOLOGIES

Cleansing is a basic skin activity resulting in the removal of sweat, sebum, bacteria, fungal elements, desquamating corneocytes, and environmental debris from the skin surface. Yet, cosmeceutical cleansers abound that require some unique consumer-perceived attribute to command a higher price. The specialty categories found in many cosmeceutical lines are discussed.

Toners

Toners, also known as astringents, are liquid cosmeceutical formulations designed for facial application in place of detergent cleansing or after detergent cleansing. Tremendous diversity in formulation abounds; however, toners work through solvency of skin soils. Cosmeceutical

Disclosure: The author has nothing to disclose.
Dermatology Consulting Services, PLLC, 2444 North Main Street, High Point, NC 27262, USA
E-mail address: zdraelos@northstate.net

Dermatol Clin 37 (2019) 107–115
https://doi.org/10.1016/j.det.2018.07.001

toner formulations are available for all skin types. Oily skin astringents contain a high concentration of alcohol, thus removing any sebum left behind after prior cleansing and producing a clean, tight feeling many consumers find desirable. Medicated astringents for acne patients may contain menthol or camphor to create a tingling feeling when applied to the skin. Astringents for normal skin contain lower alcohol concentrations whereas those for dry skin are labeled alcohol-free. Dry skin formulations contain largely propylene glycol and water to act as a humectant moisturizer.[1]

Specialty toners to enhance exfoliation may contain α-hydroxy acids, such as glycolic acid. Glycolic acid is the smallest α-hydroxy acid appearing as a colorless, odorless, hygroscopic crystalline solid. Although glycolic acid can be obtained from the fermentation of sugar cane, for cosmeceutical use it is more commonly synthesized by reacting chloroacetic acid with sodium hydroxide followed by reacidification. Another cosmeceutical toner variant is a 2-phase toner, which consists of a solvent and immiscible oil. The product is shaken prior to use to temporary emulsify the solvent and oil prior to facial application, creating unusual visual effects. Some high-end 2-phase toners even contain suspended gold leaf. Here the solvent dissolves the skin soils while the oil leaves behind a moisturizing film for amelioration of dry skin.

If a good cleanser is selected, it is not necessary to incorporate a toner into a cosmeceutical skin treatment regimen. Thus, toners are optional and not functionally necessary cosmeceuticals.

Cleansing Scrubs

Cleansing scrubs are a common part of the cosmeceutical cleansing routine used for cleansing and exfoliation purposes. The formulation contains particulates and surfactants designed to mechanically exfoliate either the face or body. Traditional surfactants are combined with aluminum oxide, ground fruit pits, polyethylene beads, or sodium tetraborate decahydrate granules to form a suspension.[2] The particles are manually massaged into the skin, dislodging desquamating corneocytes and improving skin visual smoothness and tactile softness, 2 important cosmeceutical function attributes. Typically, the scrub is used once weekly; however, more frequent or aggressive use can cause skin barrier damage and skin sensitivity. Aluminum oxide and ground fruit pits produce the most aggressive exfoliation due to their rough surface contour; however, recently, ground apricot pit powder has been introduced, producing less skin trauma.

Polyethylene beads are smooth and roll when rubbed over the skin surface, creating a milder exfoliation with little potential for skin damage; however, there are mounting environmental concerns regarding their use, with several states, such as Illinois and New York, taking steps to ban polyethylene bead–containing products.[3] After cleansing, the polyethylene beads are washed down the drain and can slip through most water treatment systems, entering the water systems of the world.[4] The microbeads soak up pollutants in the water and are eaten by fish, allowing transfer to humans of toxins, such as pesticides, flame-retardants, motor oil, and so forth.[5,6]

The use of a cleansing scrub can add to skin luminosity and radiance, 2 common cosmeceutical marketing claims. The scrubs achieve this claim by literally sanding the skin surface smooth, which increases light reflection from the skin surface, providing the physical attribute that consumers identify as luminosity and radiance. Thus, cleansing scrubs produce noticeable tangible real improvement but must be used continuously to maintain the temporary benefit.

Cleansing Cloths

Cleansing cloths are another cosmeceutical technique whereby cleansing and chemical and physical exfoliation are combined. The surfactant is impregnated in the cloth, which can be either wet or dry. The premoistened cloths are removed from the container and rubbed over the face followed by water rinsing whereas the dry cloths are moistened with water prior to use. The cloths are single use and manufactured from polyester, rayon, cotton, and cellulose fibers formed into a thin sheet via heat through a technique known as thermobonding. The fibers are further strengthened by hydroentangling, which entwines the individual rayon, polyester, and cellulose fibers with high-pressure jets of water. Further cleansing attributes are imparted by texturing the cloth with an open or closed weave. Open-weave cloths possess 2-mm to 3-mm windows between the adjacent fiber bundles, providing milder exfoliation whereas closed-weave cloths have a tighter weave and are designed to optimize removal of sebum, cosmetics, and environmental dirt while providing a more aggressive exfoliant effect. Thus, the degree of exfoliation and cleansing is dependent on cloth weave, cleansing pressure, and length of cloth cleansing time (**Fig. 1**).

The cleansing cloths can be customized for normal to oily skin, normal to dry skin, or sensitive skin. This is accomplished by modifying the sebum removal ability of the surfactant in the cloth and

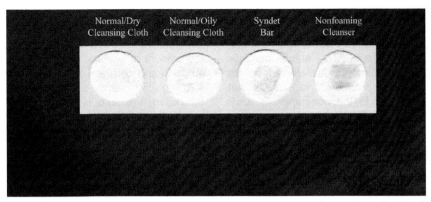

Fig. 1. Cleansing cloth efficacy. The efficacy of a cleanser can be determined by washing the facial foundation–covered face followed by wiping with a cotton pad soaked in isopropyl alcohol. The amount of colored cosmetic on the pad remained on the face after cleansing. The cleansing cloths leave behind less cosmetic than either the syndet bar cleanser or the nonfoaming cleanser, thus producing more thorough facial cleansing.

designing the weave to produce more or less exfoliation, with more exfoliation found in normal to oily skin cloths and less found in dry/sensitive skin cloths. The cleansing cloths produce real and perceived cosmeceutical benefit by smoothing the skin surface and providing enhanced cleansing by more thoroughly traversing the skin dermatoglyphics. This leads again to smoother, softer, shinier skin, which is perceived by the consumer as healthier skin.

Mechanized and Unmechanized Cleansing Brushes and Implements

Enhanced cleansing is an excellent way to produce noticeable cosmeceutical benefit within a commonly practiced daily event. Instead of using a mundane washcloth or the hands, elaborate cleansing implements can add an air of cosmeceutical sophistication to the facial cleansing ritual. These devices can be unmechanized or mechanized. The unmechanized devices can be bristled brushes, silicone cleansing pads, natural sponges, or plastic spatulas. The user applies a surfactant to the skin and then uses a hand to apply pressure and direct the implement over the skin surface. These devices produce mechanical exfoliation whereas a cleanser produces chemical exfoliation.

Recently, mechanized brushes and silicone pads have become more popular, adapting the concepts and designs found in electric toothbrushes to facial cleansing. Theoretically, these devices produce more thorough removal of skin soils than washcloth or hand cleansing. This, however, is highly device dependent. The most common mechanized brushes rotate either clockwise or counterclockwise, sweeping the bristles over the skin unidirectionally. Theoretically, better cleansing could be achieved by an oscillatory motion of the brush sweeping the bristles back and forth over the skin. One currently popular brush uses a sonicating oscillatory motion building on the skin's elastic properties to effect facial cleansing without exceeding its physical limits by use of an optimal amplitude and frequency range.[7] The differential motion applied to the skin creates a force that opens the pores to loosen and dislodge comedonal plugs and skin soil, without damaging the skin.[8]

Another recently marketed cleansing device sonicates a silicone pad that not only stretches the skin but also stretches and compresses the skin based on the friction created between the silicone fingers and the skin. This skin stretching and compressing are theorized to produce alternate-direction skin fibroblast movement, resulting in improved skin collagen. The idea is similar to the fibroblast extension observed with dermal hyaluronic acid skin fillers.

Mechanized and unmechanized cosmeceutical cleansing implements may induce enhanced skin benefits over just using a washcloth, but this is highly user and device dependent. The benefits observed with these devices are similar to the cleansing scrubs and cleansing cloths but may be superior, and the movement and pressure can be standardized. It is also possible that these devices encourage better consumer compliance with an exfoliating cleansing routine that more thoroughly traverses the skin dermatoglyphics. Nevertheless, device cleansing induces exfoliation, which is one of the tangible cosmeceutical benefits common to many cleansing regimens.

Medicated Cleansers

Many cosmeceutical lines are introducing medicated cleansers for patients with acne, based on monographed acne ingredients, such as benzoyl peroxide and salicylic acid.[9,10] This trend increased when 5% benzoyl peroxide was transferred to over-the-counter (OTC) status, because cosmeceutical manufacturers are always looking for prescription-type products and benefits that can be sold directly to the consumer. Benzoyl peroxide possesses antibacterial and comedolytic benefits and can suppress the development of resistant acne organisms when used in cleanser form.[11,12] Salicylic acid is also used as an active ingredient in OTC acne cleansers in concentrations up to 2%.[13] Salicylic acid is a colorless, crystalline, oil-soluble phenolic compound originally derived from the willow tree *Salix*, able to penetrate into the follicle and dislodge the comedonal plug from the follicular lining; however, it is not clear if these benefits are seen with short salicylic acid contact from cleansers. Salicylic acid does not kill *Propionibacterium acnes* and does not prevent the development of antibiotic resistance; however, a 2% salicylic acid scrub has demonstrated a reduction in open comedones.[14,15]

Medicated acne cleansers are now found in cosmeceutical lines for adolescents and for adults with mature hormonal acne. This concept of providing acne treatment has extended the cosmeceutical concept beyond traditional antiaging targets to targets associated with disease and problem skin. This adds more credence to the marketing idea that cosmeceuticals actually do something beyond cosmetics, which gives creditability to the brand. Thus, providing monographed acne ingredients in a more cosmetically elegant form than prescription drugs might improve compliance, consumer acceptance, and efficacy.

CLEANSER MILDNESS EVALUATION

The most important consideration in cosmeceutical cleansers is mildness. A cleanser must find a balance between removing skin soils for hygiene purposes and minimizing skin barrier damage. Usually, a new cleanser formulation is first tested in vitro followed by in vivo and Human use testing prior to marketing, because it can be difficult to predict cleanser/skin reactions.[16] The most commonly used in vitro screening tests to evaluate the irritant potential of cleansers are the collagen swelling test,[17] pH rise test,[18] and zein test.[19] Cosmeceutical manufacturers generally perform more testing of their products than usual to allow the substantiation of more robust claims and give the aura of scientific development.

One commonly used irritation test is the collagen swelling test using a 1-cm^2 collagen sheet, which is incubated for 24 hours at 50°C with a solution of the finished cleanser product at 1% of the dry extract at its own pH. The collagen is weighed before and after exposure to determine the amount of swelling associated with water absorption and collagen denaturation. More protein swelling may indicate more product irritation and the collagen exhibits surfactant damage. Another approach to irritation assessment is to examine pH rise by incubating equal volumes of a 2% solution of bovine serum albumin at a pH of 5.6 with a 2% solution of the finished product at room temperature for 1 hour. The pH of the solution is measured with greater pH rises, due to the alkaline nature of the cleanser surfactant, indicating increased product irritation. The last method, or the zein test, uses a protein that is insoluble in aqueous solution until denatured by irritating surfactant products. The more protein that is solubilized, the more irritating the product. Successful mildness determination with in vitro testing is followed-up by actual human use testing.

Many human research testing methodologies have been developed to predict the consumer response to cleansers; however, long-term use testing is clearly the most definitive.[20–22] The most commonly used in vivo method is the forearm controlled application technique (FCAT), with each company having its own internal testing standards.[23] The testing methodology is outlined in **Box 1**. This test controls the amount of cleanser applied, the length of cleansing, and the frequency of testing. It is an exaggerated use test because cleansing is performed twice daily for a 4-day test period. If a new cleanser formulation passes the in vitro and FCAT tests, it is then put into actual use testing in a wider population, sometimes composed of persons with sensitive skin or skin disease. This type of testing allows cosmeceutical manufacturers to make the following claims: mildness tested, dermatologist tested, quality tested, suitable for sensitive skin, and so forth.

COSMECEUTICAL MOISTURIZERS

Moisturizers are a key component of every cosmeceutical regimen, providing reduced transepidermal water loss that results in skin with fewer fine lines of dehydration, coats the skin with friction-reducing substances accounting for skin smoothness, and places a fine film of light-reflecting particles on the skin surface to increase radiance and luminosity. Although these are important appearance and tactile benefits, they are temporary, requiring continued use of the moisturizer to maintain the effect. Cosmeceutical manufacturers desire to create products with long-lasting benefits, such as those listed in **Box 2**. These are

Box 1
Forearm controlled application technique

1. The subject wets the left forearm with warm (90°F–100°F) tap water.
2. A wash technician wets a piece of soft towel with warm water and then squeezes the towel gently to remove excess water.
3. The moistened towel is rubbed in a circular motion on a wetted test bar for 6 seconds to generate lather.
4. The technician rubs the lathered towel in a circular motion on the application area nearest the elbow for 10 seconds.
5. The lather remains on the application area for 90 seconds.
6. The application area is rinsed with warm tap water for 15 seconds.
7. The procedure is repeated for each test product site on the left forearm.
8. The arm is patted dry.
9. The procedure is repeated for additional test sites on the right forearm.
10. After both arms have been washed once, each treatment is applied a second time for a total of 2 washes per site per visit.
11. Controlled washes are performed twice daily for 4 days spaced by a minimum of 3 hours.

Box 2
Active skin care mechanisms of action

1. Modify skin barrier
   a. Smooth skin scale
   b. Exfoliate skin scale
2. Enhance intercellular lipids
   a. Cholesterol
   b. Triglycerides
   c. Essential fatty acids
   d. Ceramides
   e. Natural moisturizing factor
3. Activate a receptor
   a. Retinoids
4. Function to protect DNA
   a. Antioxidants
   b. Sunscreens
5. Modulate a pathway
   a. Peptides
6. Activate or inhibit an enzyme
   a. Skin-lightening agents
7. Reduce inflammation
   a. Botanic antioxidants
   b. Plant sterols
8. Alter hormone balance
   a. Soy phytoestrogens

achieved through the addition of nondrug substances designed to modify the appearance of wrinkles/fine lines and skin dyspigmentation. A cosmeceutical cannot treat or eliminate any aspect of skin physiology or it is considered a drug; thus, all cosmeceutical moisturizers claim to simply modify appearance. Some of the currently popular concepts in cosmeceutical moisturizers are discussed.

Skin-Lightening Cosmeceutical Moisturizers

Skin-lightening cosmeceutical moisturizers are popular because facial dyspigmentation is universally associated with photoaging. Hydroquinone has long been the gold standard for skin lightening; however, it has become a controversial ingredient as of late. Although 4% hydroquinone falls in the pharmaceutical realm, 2% hydroquinone predated the Food and Drug Administration and remains in the cosmetic realm. It is currently under review for removal from the OTC market, encouraging many cosmeceutical manufacturers to search for alternatives. Alternatives are typically taken from the botanic and vitamin realms, because these ingredients are nonprescription, unregulated, and possess established safety profiles. Addition of skin-lightening benefits to a cosmeceutical moisturizer allows for expanded claims and enhanced scientific credibility because the "active ingredient" is assumed important and functional.

The most commonly used active ingredient for skin lightening in the current marketplace is licorice extract, known as liquiritin and isoliquertin, which are glycosides containing flavenoids.[24] Liquiritin in vitro induces skin lightening by dispersing melanin. The second most common cosmeceutical skin-lightening agent is kojic acid, chemically known as 5-hydroxymethyl-4H-pyran-4-one. It is a hydrophilic fungal derivative obtained from *Aspergillus* and *Penicillium* species.[25] The activity of kojic acid is attributed to its ability to prevent tyrosinase activity by binding to copper.[26]

Two other pigment-lightening cosmeceutical ingredients are aloesin and arbutin. Aloesin is a low-molecular-weight glycoprotein obtained from the aloe vera plant. It is a natural hydroxymethylchromone functioning to inhibit tyrosinase by competitive inhibition at the DOPA oxidation site.[27,28] It is sometimes mixed with arbutin, obtained from the leaves of the *Vaccinium vitis-idaea* plant, which is a naturally occurring glucopyranoside that causes decreased tyrosinase activity without affecting messenger RNA expression and inhibits melanosome maturation in vitro.[29]

Finally, vitamin C is used in some cosmeceutical formulations as a pigment-lightening active ingredient for its ability to interrupt melanin production by interacting with copper ions to reduce dopaquinone and blocking dihydrochinindol-2-carboxyl acid oxidation.[30] The concentration of vitamin C must be relatively low, however, because it can easily lower pH and cause cutaneous irritation.[31]

Many cosmeceutical skin-lightening preparations claim to improve the appearance of brown spots. This does not necessarily mean that the dyspigmentation is gone. The ability of a cosmeceutical to lighten skin must be evaluated on product-by-product basis. Some may have been clinically tested to demonstrate efficacy whereas others may make soft claims based on including a certain ingredient. The efficacy of cosmeceuticals cannot be guaranteed, meaning skin lighteners may or may not be of real consumer value beyond their moisturizing vehicle.

Cosmeceutical Peptide-Containing Moisturizers

Peptides are another active ingredient found in many mass market and boutique cosmeceutical lines; they are composed of amino acids, the building blocks of proteins. These are safe ingredients to include in formulations because they are foods. Peptides have been developed from raw material supplies for manufacturers to place in cosmeceutical formulations, functioning as cellular messengers, allowing receptor modulation, activating enzyme release, and regulating the production of proteins. Peptides belong to the following functional families: carrier peptides, signal peptides, and neurotransmitter peptides.[32]

Carrier peptides

The first commercialized peptides were carrier peptides designed to hook to another ingredient and facilitate transportation of the agent to the active site.[33] The first carrier peptide, GHK-Cu, was designed to deliver copper, a trace element necessary for wound healing.[34] GHK, composed of glycine, histidyl, and lysine, was originally isolated from human plasma and the synthetically

engineered. GHK-Cu was commercialized into a line of skin care products to minimize the appearance of fine lines and wrinkles based on the in vitro observation of dermal keratinocytes proliferation induction. It is hard to know, however, if the same carrier peptide result can be achieved when applying a cosmeceutical product to intact instead of wounded skin.

Signal peptides

Signal peptides are the most commonly used peptide family in cosmeceuticals. Signal peptides are designed in vitro to increase collagen, elastin, fibronectin, proteoglycan, and glycosaminoglycan production.[35] The most popular signal peptide is palmitoyl pentapeptide (Pal-KTTKS), composed of the amino acids lysine, threonine, threonine, lysine, and serine. It is a procollagen I fragment demonstrated to stimulate the production of collagen I, collagen III, and collagen IV in vitro.[36] It is used in a low concentration of 4 parts per million, because it theoretically acts as a signal whereby 1 molecule has a cascading effect. The idea is to present the body with procollagen fragments that down-regulate the production of collagenase, thereby increasing dermal collagen. This is a tremendous physiologic challenge and it is uncertain how effectively this mechanism of action works in vivo.

Neurotransmitter peptides

Neurotransmitter peptides are purported to function by inhibiting the release of acetylcholine at the neuromuscular junction. They are similar to botulinum toxin in that both selectively modulate synaptosome-associated protein (SNAP) of 25,000 Da (SNAP-25). Botulinum toxin A proteolytically degrades SNAP-25 whereas acetyl hexapeptide-3, a neurotransmitter peptide, mimics the N-terminal end of the SNAP-25 protein that inhibits the soluble N-ethylmaleimide–sensitive factor attachment protein receptor (SNARE) complex formation.[37] Acetyl hexapeptide-3, the most widely commercialized neurotransmitter peptide, inhibits vesicle docking in vitro through prevention of the SNARE complex formation, inducing muscle relaxation. This is challenging in vivo, however, because the prevention of the SNARE complex formation requires the ability to reach the neuromuscular junction molecularly intact with sufficient concentration to maintain the duration of effect.

Cosmeceutical Vitamin-Containing Moisturizers

Vitamins are commonly used active ingredients in cosmeceutical moisturizers because they are consumed foods and considered safe yet have tremendous consumer appeal.[38] The concept that skin can be nourished topically is inviting, but not physiologically relevant. Vitamins are best consumed orally and possess limited value when applied topically. Vitamins A, C, E, and B$_3$ are those most commonly selected for cosmeceutical formulation inclusion.

Vitamin A (retinoids)

Topical cosmeceutical retinoids are synthetic vitamin A derivatives, which include retinol (vitamin A alcohol), retinyl esters, retinoic acid (tretinoin), and retinyl palmitate. Retinoids are biologic modifiers producing receptor specific effects, including regulating growth of epidermal cells and promoting differentiation of cell lines.[39,40] They are difficult to topically formulate due to their inherent photo instability and degradation on exposure to oxygen.

Retinyl palmitate is the most stable of the vitamin A esters and can be easily incorporated into the oil phase of creams and lotions, due to its lipophilic nature; however, it is not very biologically active.[41] Topical activity of retinyl palmitate is believed to occur after cutaneous enzymatic cleavage of the ester bond and subsequent conversion of retinol to retinoic acid. It is this cutaneous conversion of retinol to retinoic acid that is responsible for the biologic activity of some of the new stabilized OTC retinol preparations. Unfortunately, only small amounts of retinol can be converted by the skin, accounting for the increased efficacy seen with prescription preparations containing retinoic acid.[42] Nevertheless, retinol is considered an efficacious cosmeceutical active ingredient used in many antiaging formulations for its retinoid effect.

Vitamin C

The active form of vitamin C is L-ascorbic acid, which is also light sensitive and oxygen sensitive, functioning as an antioxidant by scavenging and quenching free radicals and by regenerating vitamin E from its radical form.[43,44] Some investigators have demonstrated enhanced cutaneous vitamin C levels after topical application of 10% L-ascorbic acid; however, this work was performed on a porcine model.[45] Other human studies have demonstrated a decrease in the minimal erythema dose and less erythema after UV-B exposure in subjects treated with topical 10% L-ascorbic acid.[46] Vitamin C has also been purported to produce lightening of skin dyspigmentation in the form of magnesium L-ascorbyl-2-phosphate.[47] Vitamin C is one of the most common vitamin additives to cosmeceutical formulations. It can provide antioxidant capabilities

to the moisturizer lipids but may not always be present in sufficient concentration or the proper chemical form to act as a physiologic skin antioxidant.

Vitamin E

Vitamin E is a lipid-soluble antioxidant, with α-tocopherol possessing greater biologic activity than γ-tocopherol. Vitamin E is naturally found in the membranes of cells and organelles, preventing oxidation of the polyunsaturated fatty acids of the phospholipids in the membranes by capturing singlet oxygen species.[48] A variety of claims have been made regarding the topical cosmeceutical effects of vitamin E on the skin, including improved moisturization, increased softness, and better smoothness. Topically applied α-tocopherol has been shown to inhibit UV-B–induced edema and erythema, conferring a SPF of 3, after multiple applications.[41] This is believed due to its ability to marginally absorb light and function as a free radical–quenching, lipid-soluble antioxidant.[49] Vitamin E is lipophilic and can be incorporated into cosmeceuticals in the form of vitamin E acetate, the stable esterified form of vitamin E, and vitamin E linoleate. It probably functions more as an emollient in most cosmeceutical formulations than an active physiologic antioxidant.

Niacin

Niacin, also found on cosmeceutical ingredient disclosures as niacinamide or nicotinic acid, is a popular ingredient around which many antiaging claims have been developed. Niacin is 1 component of the B vitamin complex, known as vitamin B$_3$. It is an important part of 2 coenzymes of intermediate metabolism, nicotinamide adenine dinucleotide and nicotinamide adenine dinucleotide phosphate. It is found in moisturizers to support a variety of cosmeceutical claims: sebum inhibition, increased epidermal lipids, reduced inflammation, increased collagen production, increased dermal elasticity, and UV protection.[50–52] Most of these claims have been demonstrated in vitro only; nevertheless, niacin-containing cosmeceuticals remain popular.

SUMMARY

Cosmeceuticals are an ever-evolving and ever-expanding category of skin care. These products captivate consumers with novel ideas for appearance improvement and entice the purchase of premium priced products. The challenge is to convince purchasers that the jar contains something worth the price. This is accomplished by including novel cleansing and moisturizing devices and ingredients that meet the innate inner need of all humans to be attractive at any age. This article evaluates the data and real value of these technologies for dermatologist.

REFERENCES

1. Wilkinson JB, Moore RJ. Astringents and skin toners. In: Harry's cosmeticology. 7th edition. New York: Chemical Publishing; 1982. p. 74–81.
2. Mills OH, Kligman AM. Evaluation of abrasives in acne therapy. Cutis 1979;23:704–5.
3. Chang M. Reducing microplastics from facial exfoliating cleansers in wastewater through treatment versus consumer product decisions. Mar Pollut Bull 2015;101(1):330–3.
4. Barnes D, Galgani F, Thompson R, et al. Accumulation and fragmentation of plastic debris in global environments. Philos Trans R Soc Lond B Biol Sci 2009; 364:1985–98.
5. Mato Y, Isobe T, Takada H, et al. Plastic resin pellets as a transport medium for toxic chemicals in the marine environment. Environ Sci Technol 2001;35(2): 318–24.
6. Fendall LS, Sewell MA. Contributing to marine pollution by washing your face: microplastics in facial cleansers. Mar Pollut Bull 2009;58(8): 1225–8.
7. Draelos ZD. Reexamining methods of facial cleansing. Cosmet Dermatol 2005;18:173–5.
8. Akridge R, Ortblad O, Henes E. Clinical efficacy of a new sonic skin care brush for facial cleansing. Poster presented at: American Academy of Dermatology 64th Annual Meeting;March 3-7,2006;San Francisco, CA. J Am Acad Dermatol 2006; 54(suppl):AB50. P417.
9. Draelos ZD. The effect of a daily facial cleanser for normal to oily skin on the skin barrier of subjects with acne. Cutis 2006;78(1 Suppl):34–40.
10. Choi YS, Suh HS, Yoon MY, et al. A study of the efficacy of cleansers for acne vulgaris. J Dermatolog Treat 2010;21(3):201–5.
11. Leyden JJ, Wortzman M, Baldwin EK. Antibiotic-resistant Propionibacterium acnes suppressed by a benzoyl peroxide cleanser 6%. Cutis 2008;82(6): 417–21.
12. Del Rosso JQ. Benzoyl peroxide cleansers for the treatment of acne vulgaris: status report on available data. Cutis 2008;82(5):336–42.
13. Eady EA, Burke BM, Pulling K, et al. The benefit of 2% salicylic acid lotion in acne. J Dermatol Ther 1996;7:93–6.
14. Chen T, Appa Y. Over-the-counter acne medications. In: Draelos ZD, Thaman LA, editors. Cosmetic formulations of skin care products. New York: Taylor & Francis; 2006. p. 251–71.
15. Pagnoni A, Chen T, Duong H, et al. Clinical evaluation of a salicylic acid containing scrub, toner, mask and regimen in reducing blackheads. 61st meeting, American Academy of Dermatology. February, 2004;Poster 61.
16. Morrison BM, Paye M. A comparison of three in vitro screening tests with an in vivo clinical test to evaluate the irritation potential of antibacterial liquid soaps. J Soc Cosmet Chem 1995;46:291–9.
17. Blake-Haskins J, Scala D, Rhein LD, et al. Predicting surfactant irritation from the swelling response of a collagen film. J Soc Cosmet Chem 1986;37: 199–210.
18. Tavss EA, Eigen E, Kligman AM. Anionic detergent-induced skin irritation and anionic detergent-induced pH rise of bovine serum albumin. J Soc Cosmet Chem 1988;39:267–72.
19. Gotte E, et al. Synthetische Tenside in medizinisch-kosmetischen Baden. Aest Medizin 1996;15: 313–20.
20. Nicholl G, Murahata R, Grove G, et al. The relative sensitivity of two arm-wash methods for evaluating the mildness of personal washing products. J Soc Cosmet Chem 1995;46:129–40.
21. Strube D, Koontz S, Murahata R. The flex wash test: a method for evaluating the mildness of personal washing products. J Soc Cosmet Chem 40:297–306.
22. Wilhelm KP, Cua BC, Wolff HW, et al. Surfactant-induced stratum corneum hydration in vivo: prediction of the irritation potential of anionic surfactants. J Invest Dermatol 1993;101(3):310–5.
23. Ertel K, Keswick B, Bryant P. A forearm controlled application technique for estimating the relative mildness of personal cleansing products. J Soc Cosmet Chem 1995;46:67–76.
24. Amer M, Metwalli M. Topical Liquiritin improves melasma. Int J Dermatol 2000;39(4):299–301.
25. Lim JT. Treatment of melasma using kojic acid in a gel containing hydroquinone and glycolic acid. Dermatol Surg 1999;25:282–4.
26. Garcia A, Fulton JE Jr. The combination of glycolic acid and hydroquinone or kojic acid for the treatment of melasma and related conditions. Dermatol Surg 1996;22(5):443–7.
27. Choi S, Lee SK, Kim JE, et al. Aloesin inhibits hyperpigmentation induced by UV radiation. Clin Exp Dermatol 2002;27:513–5.
28. Jones K, Hughes J, Hong M, et al. Modulation of melanogenesis by aloesin: a competitive inhibitor of tyrosinase. Pigment Cell Res 2002;15:335–40.
29. Hori I, Nihei K, Kubo I. Structural criteria for depigmenting mechanism of arbutin. Phytother Res 2004;18:475–9.
30. Espinal-Perez LE, Moncada B, Castanedo-Cazares JP. A double blind randomized trial of 5% ascorbic acid vs 4% hydroquinone in melasma. Int J Dermatol 2004;43(8):604–7.

31. Herndon JH, Jiang LI, Kononov T, et al. An open la-bel clinical trial to evaluate the efficacy and toler-ance of a retinol and vitamin c facial regimen in women with mild-to-moderate hyperpigmentation and photodamaged facial skin. J Drugs Dermatol 2016;15(4):476–82.

32. Litner K. Peptides, amino acids and proteins in skin care? Cosmet Toilet 2007;122:26–34.

33. Gruchlik A, Jurzak M, Chodurek E, et al. Effect of Gly-Gly-His, Gly-His-Lys and their copper com-plexes on TNF-alpha-dependent IL-6 secretion in normal human dermal fibroblasts. Acta Pol Pharm 2012;69(6):1303–6.

34. Maquart FX, Pickart L, Laurent M, et al. Stimulation of collagen synthesis in fibroblast cultures by the tripepetide-copper complex glycyl-L-histidyl-L-Cu^{2+}. FEBS Lett 1988;238:343–5.

35. Zhang L, Falla TJ. Cosmeceuticals and peptides. Clin Dermatol 2009;27(5):485–94.

36. Katayama K, Armendariz-Borunda J, Raghow R, et al. A pentapeptide from type I procollagen pro-motes extracellular matrix production. J Biol Chem 1993;268:9941–4.

37. Blanes-Mira C, Cemente J, Jodas G, et al. A synthetic hexapeptide (Argireline) with antiwrinkle activity. Int J Cosmet Sci 2002;24:303–10.

38. Manela-Azulay M, Bagatin E. Cosmeceuticals vita-mins. Clin Dermatol 2009;27(5):469–74.

39. Goodman DS. Vitamin A and retinoids in health and disease. N Engl J Med 1984;310(16):1023–31.

40. Noy N. Interactions of retinoids with lipid bilayers and with membranes. In: Livrea MA, Packer L, edi-tors. Retinoids. New York: Marcel Dekker; 1993. p. 17–27.

41. Idson B. Vitamins and the skin. Cosmet Toilet 1993; 108:79–92.

42. Babamiri K, Nassab R. Cosmeceuticals: the evi-dence behind the retinoids. Aesthet Surg J 2010; 30(1):74–7.

43. Chan AC. Partners in defense, vitamin E, and vitamin C. Can J Physiol Pharmacol 1993;71: 725–31.

44. Beyer RE. The role of ascorbate in antioxidant pro-tection of biomembranes: interaction with vitamin E and coenzyme Q. J Bioenerg Biomembr 1994;26: 349–58.

45. Darr D, Combs S, Dunston S, et al. Topical vitamin C protects procine shin from ultraviolet radiation-induced damage. Br J Dermatol 1992;127:247–53.

46. Murray J, Darr D, Reich J, et al. Topical vitamin C treatment reduces ultraviolet B radiation-induced er-ythema in human skin (abstract). J Invest Dermatol 1991;96:587.

47. Kameyama K, Sakai C, Kondoh S, et al. Inhibitory ef-fects of magnesium L-ascorbyl-2-phosphate on melanogenesis in vitro and in vivo. J Am Acad Der-matol 1996;34:29–33.

48. Burton GW, Joyce A, Ingold KU. Is vitamin E the only lipid-soluble, chain-breaking antioxidant in human blood plasma and erythrocyte membranes? Arch Biochem Biophys 1983;221:281–90.

49. Mayer P, Pittermann W, Wallat S. The effects of vitamin E on the skin. Cosmet Toilet 1993;108: 99–109.

50. Bissett DL, Miyamoto K, Sun P, et al. Topical niacin-amide reduces yellowing, wrinkling, red blotchiness, and hyperpigmented spots in aging facial skin. Int J Cosmet Sci 2004;26:231–8.

51. Bissett DL, Oblong JE, Saud A, et al. Topical niacin-amide provides skin aging appearance benefits while enhancing barrier function. J Clin Dermatol 2003;32S:9–18.

52. Farris P, Zeichner J, Berson D. Efficacy and tolera-bility of a skin brightening/anti-aging cosmeceutical containing retinol 0.5%, niacinamide, hexylresorcin-ol, and resveratrol. J Drugs Dermatol 2016;15(7): 863–8.

What's New in Cosmetic Dermatology

Anthony V. Benedetto, DO[a,b],*

KEYWORDS

- Topical silicone gel • Topical triple antibiotic ointment • Vaginal laser rejuvenation
- Genitourinary syndrome of menopause • Botulinum toxins • OnabotulinumtoxinA
- DaxibotulinumtoxinA

KEY POINTS

- Topical silicone gel is preferred over petrolatum-based products as an all-purpose wound dressing for granulating and sutured wounds, regardless of cause.
- Vaginal laser rejuvenation is effective in relieving genitourinary syndrome of menopause (GSM), stress urinary incontinence (SUI), vaginal relaxation syndrome (VRS), vulvar disorders of lichen sclerosis, and other related issues.
- New cosmetic indications in the upper face for onabotulinumtoxinA have been approved by the FDA and off-label treatments for the lower face are increasing in popularity.
- Clinical trials of uncomplicated daxibotulinumtoxinA demonstrate safety and efficacy lasting more than six months.

TOPICAL SILICONE VERSUS PETROLATUM-BASED PRODUCTS AS A PREFERRED POSTSURGICAL WOUND DRESSING

The use of topical antibiotics after dermatologic surgical procedures has always been controversial in preventing surgical site infections. In the United States, dermatologists perform more than 25 million procedures yearly that result in superficial cutaneous wounds, which are low risk for postoperative infection.[1] The ever-growing routine use of topical antibiotics is unnecessary and currently not recommended. Because there is no scientific proof that the application of topical antibiotics onto a wound bed after cutaneous surgery prevents surgical site infections, the use of topical antibiotics postoperatively has become a habit without evidence.[2] This practice potentially places patients at risk for allergic or irritant contact dermatitis, contributes to delayed wound healing, produces multidrug-resistant bacterial infections, and even contributes to inflammatory chondritis and anaphylaxis.[3] Therefore, the current recommendations for wound care are to limit the use of topical antibiotics to avoid the ever-increasing incidence of bacterial resistance.[1–6] Reconsideration of the standards for postoperative wound care is highly recommended and necessary. Recently, a one question survey by the author was conducted of prospective patients presenting to a dermatologic surgical practice. (Staidle JP, Benedetto AV, Benedetto PX, et al. Comparison of a novel antibiotic-free film-forming topical wound dressing versus triple antibiotic on Mohs surgical wounds. Submitted for publication.) Before the patients were seen by their dermatologist, they were asked to respond to this question: "What is your favorite 'go to' over the counter first aid cream or ointment that you use to help heal a scratch, cut or burn?" Nearly 82% of the more than 960 responders indicated that they prefer a topical petrolatum-

Disclosure: The author has nothing to disclose.
[a] Department of Dermatology, Perelman School of Medicine, University of Pennsylvania, 3400 Civic Center Boulevard, Philadelphia, PA 19104, USA; [b] Dermatologic SurgiCenter, 1200 Locust Street, Philadelphia, PA 19107, USA
* Corresponding author. Department of Dermatology, Perelman School of Medicine, University of Pennsylvania, 3400 Civic Center Boulevard, Philadelphia, PA 19104, USA.
E-mail address: avb@benedettoderm.com

Dermatol Clin 37 (2019) 117–128
https://doi.org/10.1016/j.det.2018.08.002
0733-8635/19/© 2018 Elsevier Inc. All rights reserved.

based product, of which more than 45% used some form of a triple antibiotic containing neomycin, bacitracin, or polymyxin B and another 25% admitted to using a topical bacitracin and polymyxin B product, and nearly 10% of the remaining responders used some form of topical petrolatum with or without an antibiotic component.

Other studies have shown topical silicone is safer and more effective as a postoperative wound dressing when compared with any petrolatum-based product with or without an antibiotic component.[8–11] The reason for this is silicone is inert and has no measurable pH. It is mostly bacteriostatic and for some bacteria it is bactericidal. However, petrolatum has a measurable pH and can promote microbial overgrowth. Topical silicone gel (SG) is nonocclusive, waterproof, and gas permeable. Petrolatum is a water immiscible, occlusive ointment and inhibits the exchange of gases (eg, oxygen and carbon dioxide) to occur freely from the surface of the wound. Petrolatum adheres to the wound bed and causes maceration, whereas silicone is a flexible hydrophobic barrier maintaining normal ambient wound hydration and decreases transepidermal water loss. Petrolatum, conversely, saturates and macerates cutaneous tissue and has no effect on a wound's transepidermal water loss. Because of its inherent properties, silicone protects open wounds from chemical and microbial invasion, reduces inflammation, and thereby lessens abnormal scar formation. Petrolatum is only partially protective of external chemical and microbial insults on open wounds, has no effect on reducing the extent of inflammation, nor does it have any effect on scar formation.

Because recent reports confirmed the benefits of using topical SG as a postoperative wound dressing,[8–11] we initiated a phase IV, postmarketing, prospective, open label trial to compare the use of topical SG (Stratamed, Stratpharma, Basel, Switzerland) against the popular and frequently used topical triple antibiotic ointment (TA) Neosporin, containing bacitracin, neomycin, and polymyxin B (Johnson &Johnson, New Brunswick,

NJ). Neosporin ointment was used in this comparative study because of its widespread and regular use by the general public and physicians alike, which was disclosed by the internal survey conducted by the author.[7] There were two arms to the study. One cohort of 60 patients underwent Mohs surgery and the postoperative wounds were dressed with either SG (n = 30) or TA (n = 30). The other cohort of 274 patients underwent general excisional surgery or a typical dermatologic surgical procedure, such as a biopsy, curettage, or even extensive cryosurgery with liquid nitrogen. The primary objectives of this clinical study were to measure the incidence of contact or irritant dermatitis, the rate of infection, healing time, and the quality of healing as assessed by the patient and a physician observer. The secondary objectives were to document the patients' comfort level with using either product, ease of dressing changes, and overall satisfaction with either product.

The Mohs surgery arm of the study has been completed.[7] None of the patients using SG developed any sign of contact or irritant dermatitis. There was a 21.6% incidence of contact or irritant dermatitis in patients using the TA. The incidence of infection was not significantly different between either group ($P > .05$). Both the healing time ($P = .018$) and healing quality ($P<.001$) were significantly better in the SG group as compared with the TA group, measured on a scale of −4 (much worse) to +4 (much better).

Fig. 1 is an example of a patient who used the SG product and **Fig. 2** is an example of a patient who used the TA product. It was found by both the patient and physician observer that with SG there usually was less inflammation during early healing and at the time of suture removal. Because of this improved healing quality and ease of use, most patients preferred the SG product over the TA product. However, most of the Mohs wound sites at 3 months had a similar aesthetic appearance whether treated with SG or TA.

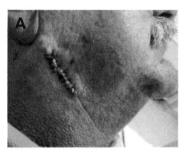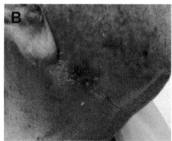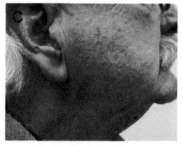

Fig. 1. This 66-year-old patient treated with silicone WD gel is shown immediately following Mohs surgery and repair (*A*), 1 week postoperatively following suture removal (*B*), and 7 months postoperatively at final assessment (*C*).

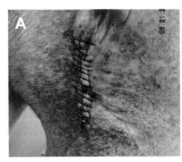
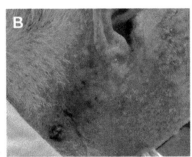
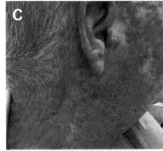

Fig. 2. This 61-year-old patient treated with TA ointment is shown immediately following Mohs surgery and repair (A), 1 week postoperatively following suture removal (B), and 7 months postoperatively at his final assessment (C). (Note the increased erythema at the time of suture removal.)

In conclusion, the SG film forming wound dressing demonstrated no contact or irritant dermatitis nor increased infection rate when compared with the TA. Wound healing quality was enhanced, and ease of use was better with the SG as compared with the petrolatum-based topical triple antibiotic. The SG used in this study is the first topical SG dressing indicated for the immediate application on granulating and sutured wounds. When used immediately after surgery it may also contribute to minimizing postoperative scar formation. Topical silicone is antibiotic free and can be used as an all-purpose alternative for routine wound care regardless of cause and should be preferred over any petrolatum-based product.

CARBON DIOXIDE LASER VAGINAL REJUVENATION

Women's health issues concerning urinary incontinence, vaginal dryness, vulvovaginal itching and burning, vaginal laxity, pain with intercourse, and sexual dysfunction recently have become frequent topics in the popular visual media and in print. Because of the widespread awareness of these overwhelming issues, vaginal rejuvenation has become a hot topic not only in the media, but also in doctors' offices. Treatments with laser and light-based devices to manage such devastating issues are on the rise, increasing at a rate of 26% annually and estimated to triple in 5 years. North America is expected to be the largest market for vaginal laser rejuvenation, predicted to expand by 30% each year through 2021. More than 500,000 feminine rejuvenation procedures were performed in 2016, and by 2021 more than 27,000 devices will be in operation.[12]

The most common condition that may affect women over a certain age is the genitourinary syndrome of menopause (GSM), which is caused by a diminution in estrogen production and secretion by the ovaries, causing atrophic vaginitis. Stress urinary incontinence, caused by a weakening in the suspension of the urinary bladder, can lead to involuntary loss of urine with minimal abrupt physical activities like coughing, laughing, walking, sitting down, or standing up. Vaginal relaxation syndrome (VRS), most commonly caused by vaginal childbirth, can affect younger and older women. Other vulvar issues of concern are certain dermatoses, such as lichen sclerosis and vulvodynia.[13]

Approximately 60% to 80% of postmenopausal women develop GSM, whose symptoms are caused by intravaginal mucosal atrophy, dryness, and inflammation, leading to vulvovaginal itching, burning, soreness, and discharge; dyspareunia, and postcoital bleeding. When this occurs more than 40% of women experience quality of life issues and some form of sexual dysfunction; 34% have arousal difficulties, 20% have lack of desire, and 19% have orgasmic dysfunction.[14] Of the women who have urinary issues, 50% are caused by stress urinary incontinence manifested by urgency, burning, with urination, and frequent urinary tract infections; another 20% are attributed to urinary urgency.

In the United States, atrophic vaginitis occurs in more than 50 million women, more commonly seen in premenopausal and postmenopausal women and even in those of child bearing age (25–50 years old). Of the women who have atrophic vaginitis, 26 million (59%) have given birth to children. Approximately 70% of the 3 million women (2.1 million) in the United States who are survivors of breast cancer have atrophic vaginitis, and approximately 300,000 new cases of breast cancer are reported in the United States annually.[15] All these women suffering from atrophic vaginitis can benefit from some form of treatment to relieve their incapacitating symptoms. Of the women who are not at risk for breast or other endocrine cancers, but have postmenopausal hormonal issues, hormone-replacement therapy is an option. However, for those women at risk, treatment with a laser or light-based device is a preferred therapeutic option.

Before menopause the ovaries produce sufficient amounts of estrogen, which maintains a thick and moist mucosal lining of the vagina, and blood flow to the vaginal tissue is abundant. Walls of the vagina are elastic and the moist mucosal surfaces secrete additional mucus during sexual activity. However, in postmenopausal women the ovaries produce little to no estrogen, causing the vaginal lining to become atrophic and dry. There is a decrease in blood flow to the vaginal tissues, resulting in a decrease in vaginal elasticity and a reduction in mucous secretion at all times, even during sexual activity. There also is a narrowing and shortening of the vaginal vault and atrophy of vulvar supportive structures.

The vaginal wall is composed of four layers: (1) a superficial layer of stratified squamous epithelium, (2) the lamina propria, (3) a fibromuscular layer, and (4) the adventitia. The stratified squamous epithelial lining of the vaginal vault provides protection against mechanical friction and is lubricated by glycogen-rich mucus. Vaginal walls do not contain any glandular structures. Estrogen stimulates the superficial and intermediate epithelial cells of the mucosal lining to secrete glycogen. In premenopausal women the superficial and intermediate cells predominate and are well-estrogenized, thick, and full of glycogen, secreting an abundance of mucus as needed. However, because of the diminution in estrogen secretion in GSM, there is a substantial reduction in the superficial cells of the epithelium and increase in parabasal and nonproductive intermediate cells (Fig. 3).

Another distressing problem for women is vaginal laxity or vaginal relaxation syndrome (VRS). The vagina can stretch up to 200% because the walls are composed of elastic soft tissue folds called rugae. VRS can occur for multiple reasons, but mostly because of multiple vaginal deliveries with or without instrumentation, advancing age, menopause, excessive sexual activity, or related trauma.[16]

Table 1 compares the different technologies of radiofrequency devices, erbium-doped:YAG lasers, and carbon dioxide (CO_2) lasers. Typically, radiofrequency treatments for vaginal rejuvenation primarily involve tissue coagulation, so therefore are somewhat painful and can take up to 30 to 45 minutes to complete. Erbium-doped:YAG lasers ablate tissue more quickly, usually within 15 minutes, but because of its high affinity for water, ablation of the vaginal mucosa is superficial. Fractional CO_2 laser treatments can take anywhere between 5 to 15 minutes to perform, depending on the proprietary laser used. Advantages of the CO_2 laser are that treatments include ablation and coagulation of the vaginal mucosa. This combined thermal effect on vaginal mucosa by CO_2 lasers can tighten vaginal laxity by improving pelvic floor support; enhance vaginal glycogen production and lubrication; and reduce symptoms of GSM, increase sexual sensation, and decrease dyspareunia. Other benefits are a reduction in stress urinary incontinence, a decrease in urinary tract infections, and symptomatic relief of lichen sclerosis and vulvodynia.

WHAT'S NEW IN THE WORLD OF THE BOTULINUM TOXINS: NEW TREATMENTS AND NEW PRODUCTS

In 2017, the Food and Drug Administration approved the cosmetic treatment of forehead

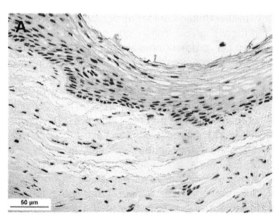
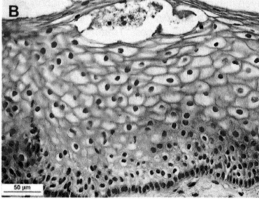

Fig. 3. Photomicrograph of a biopsy of an atrophic vaginal wall before treatment (A) and after the third treatment (B) with CO_2 laser of the same patient. Note the increase in glycogen-filled intermediate cells of the vaginal epithelium (H&E, original magnification ×40).

Table 1
A comparison of the different technologies of radiofrequency, erbium-doped:YAG and fractional CO_2 lasers

Technology	Mechanism	Procedural Time
Radiofrequency (ThermiVa; Viveve Cryo MonoRF)	Transmucosal heating tissue to 40°C–45°C, promotes prolonged edema	Up to 30 min (internal), 45 min (external) per area; multiple treatments required
Erbium-doped:YAG (Diva)	Collagen contracture from wound healing response	15–20 min; minimal thermal effect; superficial ablation
Fractional CO_2 (radiofrequency excited) super pulse only capability (FemiLift; MonaLisaTouch; Intima; GyneLase)	Ablation + coagulation induced collagen contraction, elastin production	10–20 min for internal treatments 10–15 min for external treatments (when available)
Fractional CO_2 (DC-excited) continuous wave and super pulse capabilities (FemTouch)	Ablation + coagulation induced collagen contraction, elastin production	3–5 min for internal treatments 5–10 min for external treatments

horizontal wrinkle lines with onabotulinumtoxinA. Now injections of onabotulinumtoxinA in the upper face with a total of 64 U placed in 16 sites is Food and Drug Administration approved (**Fig. 4**). Injecting forehead horizontal lines is approved for 20 U of onabotulinumtoxinA placed in five sites. Injecting glabella lines is approved for 20 U injected in five sites and lateral canthal lines is approved for 24 U in six sites.

Off-label treatments of botulinum toxin type A (BoNT-A) recently have become more popular, especially in the lower face. When treating the lower face with botulinum toxin, one must consider the directional movements of not only the levators and depressors of the lower face but also those of the platysma. The platysma has three portions (pars mandibularis, pars labialis, and pars modiolaris), which collectively interdigitate with all the peribuccal levators and depressors of the lower face (**Fig. 5**). By treating the lower face as one cosmetic unit,[17,18] a balanced and natural-appearing enhancement of the lower face is achieved. These treatments include injecting the orbicularis oris to diminish perioral vertical lip lines, the depressor anguli oris for lifting down-turned oral commissures and reducing marionette lines, and the mentalis for effacing corrugated chin lines. Direct and deliberate injections of the platysma

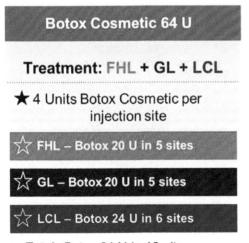

Botox Cosmetic 64 U

Treatment: FHL + GL + LCL

★ 4 Units Botox Cosmetic per injection site

☆ FHL – Botox 20 U in 5 sites

☆ GL – Botox 20 U in 5 sites

☆ LCL – Botox 24 U in 6 sites

• **Total:** Botox 64 U in 16 sites

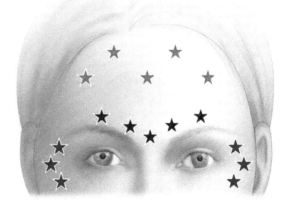

Fig. 4. Note the pattern of injections and number of units of onabotulinumtoxinA that are Food and Drug Administration approved for the cosmetic treatment of upper face wrinkles. Each star represents 4 U of onabotulinumtoxinA. FHL, forehead horizontal lines; GL, glabella lines; LCL, lateral canthal lines.

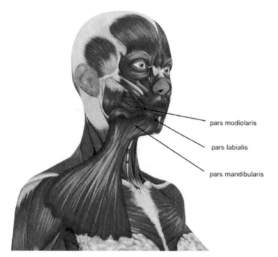

pars modiolaris

pars labialis

pars mandibularis

Fig. 5. Note the location of the platysma and its three portions in the lower face. (*Copyright 2018 From* Benedetto AV. Cosmetic uses of botulinum toxin A in the lower face, neck, and upper chest. In: Benedetto AV, ed. Botulinum Toxins in Clinical Aesthetic Practice Volume Two: Functional Anatomy and Injection Techniques. 3rd ed, Boca Raton: CRC Press, 2018:275; with permission. Reproduced by permission of Taylor and Francis Group, LLC, a division of Informa plc.)

itself in different locations in the lower face and neck with BoNT-A can attenuate lower face rhytides, soften platysmal bands, and diminish horizontal neck lines. They also can eliminate wrinkling of the décolleté and uplift breasts.[17] **Figs. 6–11** illustrate the pretreatment conditions and post-treatment results of injecting onabotulinumtoxinA in the lower face musculature, including the platysma.

In 2015, the worldwide neurotoxin market reached $3.4 billion. It is expected to grow at an annual growth rate of 8% to reach $7.3 billion in 2025.[19] This escalation in treatments is attributed to the growing popularity of minimally invasive cosmetic treatments in India, China, South Korea, Japan, and other Asian Pacific countries.[20] Competition within the neurotoxin market is increasing not only in the West with Allergan, Galderma, Merz, and Revance, but also in Asia with Medytox, Lanzhou, Daewoong, Hugel, and other manufacturers and distributors based in China, Japan, and South Korea. **Table 2** identifies the major brands of botulinum toxin available worldwide for aesthetic use. **Table 3** identifies the different companies worldwide that are in the process of developing topical botulinum toxin products. **Table 4** identifies the approved BoNT products from Asia as of early 2017. Medytox, Inc is the only biopharmaceutical company in the world to have three different physical forms of botulinumtoxinA: Neuronox (900 kDa), a complexed BoNT-A; INNOTOX (900 kDa), the world's first liquid formulation of BTX-A; and Coretox (150 kDa), a noncomplexed BoNT-A. In 2013, Medytox, Inc sold to Allegan the worldwide rights to INNOTOX, a liquid BoNT-A, but still retains the rights to sell INNOTOX in Korea. Allergan is scheduled to begin phase III trials of INNOTOX shortly.

A privately held biotechnology company, Bonti, Inc (Newport Beach, CA) is in phase 2 trials evaluating a short-acting botulinum toxin type E (BoNT-E), which has a fast onset of action of about 24 hours and a short duration of effect of about 2 to 4 weeks. Their aesthetic BoNT-E product (EB-001A) is being developed to treat glabellar frown lines, and to reduce scarring at excision sites

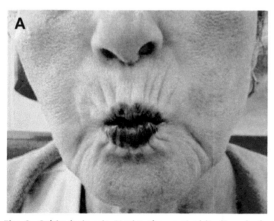
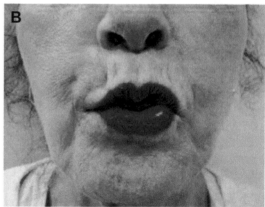

Fig. 6. Orbicularis oris. Notice the vertical lip lines before treatment (*A*) and their reduction and eversion of the vermillion with lip puckering 3 weeks after (*B*) injections of BoNT-A. (*Copyright 2018 From* Benedetto AV. Cosmetic uses of botulinum toxin A in the lower face, neck, and upper chest. In: Benedetto AV, ed. Botulinum Toxins in Clinical Aesthetic Practice Volume Two: Functional Anatomy and Injection Techniques. 3rd ed, Boca Raton: CRC Press, 2018: 249; with permission. Reproduced by permission of Taylor and Francis Group, LLC, a division of Informa plc.)

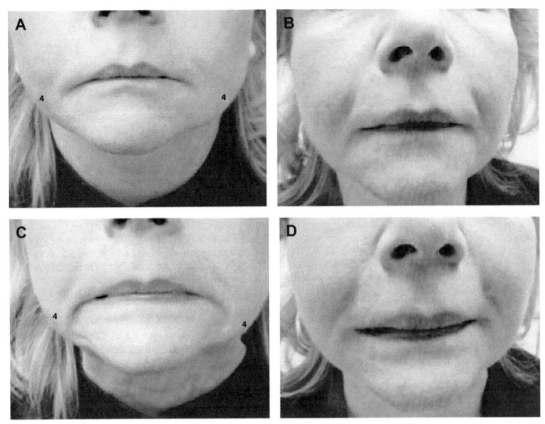

Fig. 7. Note the down-turned commissures and deep marionette lines in this 52-year-old patient at rest and with forced frowning before treatment (*A, C*) and the reduction in the down-turned commissures and diminution of marionette lines 3 weeks after (*B, D*) injections of onabotulinumtoxinA in the depressor anguli oris. (*Copyright 2018 From* Benedetto AV. Cosmetic uses of botulinum toxin A in the lower face, neck, and upper chest. In: Benedetto AV, ed. Botulinum Toxins in Clinical Aesthetic Practice Volume Two: Functional Anatomy and Injection Techniques. 3rd ed, Boca Raton: CRC Press, 2018: 263; with permission. Reproduced by permission of Taylor and Francis Group, LLC, a division of Informa plc.)

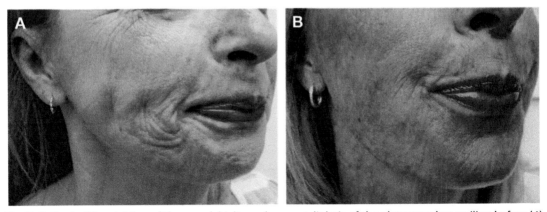

Fig. 8. Patient with wrinkling of the, pars labialis, and pars modiolaris of the platysma when smiling before (*A*) and 3 weeks after (*B*) an injection of onabotulinumtoxinA. (*Copyright 2018 From* Benedetto AV. Cosmetic uses of botulinum toxin A in the lower face, neck, and upper chest. In: Benedetto AV, ed. Botulinum Toxins in Clinical Aesthetic Practice Volume Two: Functional Anatomy and Injection Techniques. 3rd ed, Boca Raton: CRC Press, 2018: 275; with permission. Reproduced by permission of Taylor and Francis Group, LLC, a division of Informa plc.)

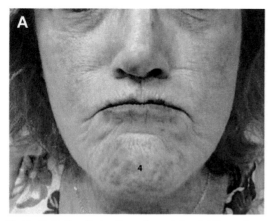
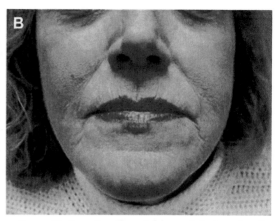

Fig. 9. Note the diminution of mental wrinkles and corrugations with the relaxation of the mentalis 6 weeks after treatment with 4 U of onabotulinumtoxinA in the center of the chin. (*Copyright 2018 From* Benedetto AV. Cosmetic uses of botulinum toxin A in the lower face, neck, and upper chest. In: Benedetto AV, ed. Botulinum Toxins in Clinical Aesthetic Practice Volume Two: Functional Anatomy and Injection Techniques. 3rd ed, Boca Raton: CRC Press, 2018: 272; with permission. Reproduced by permission of Taylor and Francis Group, LLC, a division of Informa plc.)

following Mohs surgery and reconstruction of head and neck skin cancers. The results of their phase 2a clinical trial of moderate to severe glabellar frown lines demonstrated a favorable safety profile while confirming the expected clinical effects. Their phase 2a SHINE-1 (Scar Healing Improvement with Neurotoxin-E) clinical trial after Mohs surgery is still underway.

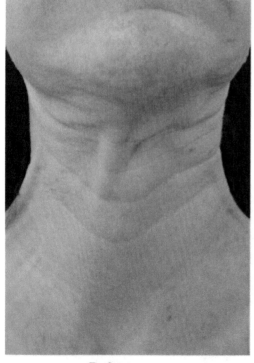
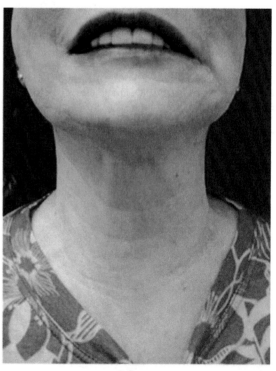

Before   After

Fig. 10. Note the diminution of platysmal bands 1 month after injections of onabotulinumtoxinA. (*Copyright 2018 From* Benedetto AV. Cosmetic uses of botulinum toxin A in the lower face, neck, and upper chest. In: Benedetto AV, ed. Botulinum Toxins in Clinical Aesthetic Practice Volume Two: Functional Anatomy and Injection Techniques. 3rd ed, Boca Raton: CRC Press, 2018: 286; with permission. Reproduced by permission of Taylor and Francis Group, LLC, a division of Informa plc.)

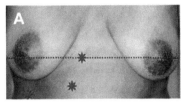
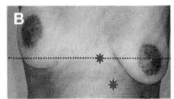
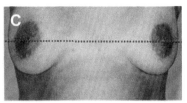

Fig. 11. Before (*A*) and 2 weeks after (*B*) 45 U of onabotulinumtoxinA injected in the right pectoralis. (*C*) One month after right pectoralis injection and 2 weeks after left pectoralis was injected with onabotulinumtoxinA. Note the 1.8-cm elevation of both breasts after treatment. (*Copyright 2018 From* Benedetto AV. Cosmetic uses of botulinum toxin A in the lower face, neck, and upper chest. In: Benedetto AV, ed. Botulinum Toxins in Clinical Aesthetic Practice Volume Two: Functional Anatomy and Injection Techniques. 3rd ed, Boca Raton: CRC Press, 2018: 296; with permission. Reproduced by permission of Taylor and Francis Group, LLC, a division of Informa plc.)

Their therapeutic product (EB-001T) is being developed to treat surgical and nonsurgical pain by decreasing muscle hyperactivity and spasms. The first of their two therapeutic clinical trials LANTERN-1 (Long-Acting NeuroToxin-E Relief, Non-opioid-1) is a placebo-controlled, double-blind, ascending dose cohort trial to evaluate the safety and efficacy of EB-001T injected intramuscularly in subjects undergoing elective augmentation mammaplasty. EB-001T showed favorable safety results and was well tolerated in a wide dose range without reaching a maximum tolerated dose. The highest EB-001T dose tested in LANTERN-1 was eight-fold higher than the maximum dose in their successful glabellar frown lines study. LANTERN-1 was pivotal in establishing a safe dose range for use in larger muscles. LANTERN-2 is a randomized, placebo-controlled, ascending dose, double-blind clinical trial to evaluate the safety and efficacy of treating focal muscle pain with a single intramuscular injection of EB-001T administered intraoperatively into the large rectus abdominis muscle in subjects undergoing elective abdominoplasty with plication of the rectus abdominis sheath. The primary end point is a reduction of postoperative pain at rest as measured by the Numeric Pain Rating Scale over the first 96 hours. Secondary end points include Numeric Pain Rating Scale scores during activity and patient use of rescue medications, including opioids, to address unrelieved pain. Bonti predicts their BoNT-E will be an effective,

Table 2
Major BoNT brands available worldwide for aesthetic use

Product	Company	Country	Bacterial Production Strain	Process	U/Vial (Product Specific)[a]	Excipients (in Vial)
Dysport/ Dyslor/ Azzalure	Ipsen/ Galderma	France/ Switzerland	Hall NCTC 2916	Precipitation, dialysis, chromatography	125/300/350	0.125 mg HSA 2.5 mg lactose
Botox/Botox Cosmetic/ Vistabel/ Vistabex/ Vista	Allergan Plc	United States/ Ireland	Hall-hyper	Acid precipitations, dialysis	50/100/200	0.5 mg HSA 0.9 mg NaCl
Xeomin/ Xeomin Cosmetic/ Bocouture	Merz GmbH	Germany	Hall ATCC 3502	Unknown	50/100/200	1 mg HSA 4.7 mg sucrose

Note: All products are either freeze dried (Dysport and Xeomin families) or vacuum-dried (Botox family).
Abbreviation: HAS, human serum albumin.
[a] The potency units of each product are specific to that product and are not interchangeable with those for other BoNT products.
Courtesy of Pickett A, PhD, Wrexham, UK.

Table 3
Topical BoNT being developed worldwide

Company	Country	Product Name	Technology	Clinical Data Published	Comments
Revance Therapeutics, Inc	United States	RT001	TransMTS	Yes	Moved RT001 into preclinical studies
Transdermal Corp	Canada	CosmeTox	InParT (mixed micelles/ionic nanoparticles	Yes	
Anterios, Inc Allergan Plc	United States	ANT-1207 Lotion	Unknown	No	Company purchased by Allergan, PLC (January 2016)
Malvern Cosmeceuticals, Ltd	UK	MCL005	Unknown	No	

Courtesy of Pickett A, PhD, Wrexham, UK.

Table 4
Approved BoNT products from Asia as of early 2017

Product	Company	Country	Bacterial Production Strain	Process	U/Vial (Product Specific)	Excipients (in vial)[a]
BTXA/ Prosigne/ Redux/ Lantox/ Lanzox	Lanzhou Institute of Biological Products/Hugh Source Int'l	China	Hall-hyper	Crystallization, dialysis	50/100 U	5 mg gelatin 25 mg dextran 25 mg sucrose
Meditoxin/ Neuronox/ Siax/ Botulift/ Cunox	Medytox Inc	South Korea	Hall-hyper	Acid precipitations, dialysis	50/100/ 200 U	0.5 mg HSA 0.9 mg NaCl
Innotox/ MT10109 L (liquid product)	Medytox Inc	South Korea	Hall-hyper	Unknown	25/50 U	No HSA or animal products
Coretox/ MT10107 (naked toxin, no neurotoxin-associated proteins)	Medytox Inc	South Korea	Hall-hyper	Unknown	100 U	Methionine; polysorbate-20; sucrose
Botulax/ Zentox/ Regenox	Hugel Pharma	South Korea	CBFC26	Protamine sulfate diethylamino-ethanol sepharose chromatography	50/100/ 200 U	0.5 mg HSA 0.9 mg NaCl
Nabota/ Evosyal (DWP 450)	Daewoong Pharamceutical Co Ltd	South Korea	Hall?	High-Pure Technology (patented)	100 U	0.5 mg HSA 0.9 mg NaCl

Abbreviation: HAS, human serum albumin.
[a] Concentrations of excipients may depend on the number of units in vial.
Courtesy of Pickett A, PhD, Wrexham, UK.

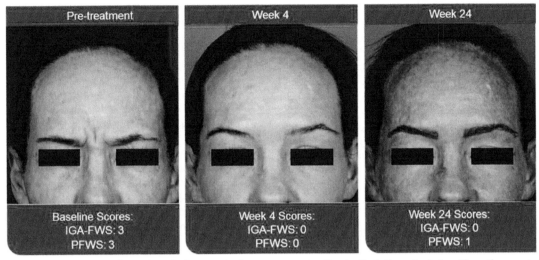

Fig. 12. A Revance study patient before and after treatment with daxibotulinumtoxinA with a three-point improvement by IGA-FWS and PFWS at Week 4 and a three-point sustained duration of effect by IGA-FWS over 24 weeks. IGA-FWS, Investigator Global Assessment Frown Wrinkle Severity; PFWS, Patient Frown Wrinkle Severity.

long-acting, nonopioid treatment of focal musculoskeletal pain, regardless of cause, which should help reduce the current demand for and abuse of opioids.

Lastly, there is a new BoNT-A under investigation for aesthetic and therapeutic use called daxibotulinumtoxinA. Produced by Revance Therapeutics (Newark, CA), it is free of accessory proteins and has a molecular weight of 150 kDa. It contains no human serum albumin or other human- or animal-derived components but contains a proprietary stabilizing excipient peptide (RTP004) that is cationic and binds to the BoNT-A molecule. Final results of their phase 3 pivotal studies, including the open label safety study, are about to be released. Preliminary results seem to indicate that patients with moderate to severe glabellar lines demonstrated a median duration of wrinkle reduction of 6 months on multiple clinically meaningful outcome measures (**Fig. 12**). Both phase 3 studies with 40 units of daxibotulinumtoxinA met their primary end point of a 2-point composite response at Week 4 and demonstrated duration of effect at more than 24 weeks. Time to return to baseline wrinkle severity, as assessed by patient and independent physician observer, exceeded 6 months and lasted up to 9 months in some subjects. Results of the clinical trials indicated that no study patient discontinued their treatment because of any adverse event.

The evolving field of cosmetic dermatology is only at the threshold of a vast array of promising innovations. Dermatologists should look to the future and eagerly embrace novel developments for the sake of improving their patients' quality of life. Reexamining antiquated therapeutic modalities is the obligation of every physician, regardless of specialty. The implementation of new treatments, such as replacing petrolatum-based products with silicone gel for more effective postoperative wound care, ablating already atrophic vaginal mucosa to regenerate glycogen-rich epithelial cells, or using a botulinum toxin to relieve pain and prevent scars, may all sound counterintuitive or even preposterous. But when evidence proves otherwise, physicians should feel reassured to incorporate such unlikely therapeutic modalities into their daily armamentarium.

REFERENCES

1. Sheth VM, Weitzul S. Postoperative topical antimicrobial use. Dermatitis 2008;19:181–9.
2. Del Rosso JQ, Kim GK. Topical antibiotics: therapeutic value or ecologic mischief? Dermatol Ther 2009;22:398–406.
3. Sachs B, Fischer-Barth W, Erdmann S, et al. Anaphylaxis and toxic epidermal necrolysis or Stevens-Johnson syndrome after nonmucosal topical drug application: fact or fiction? Allergy 2007;62:877–83.
4. Alanis AJ. Resistance to antibiotics: are we in the post-antibiotic era? Arch Med Res 2005;36: 697–705.
5. Brian MJ. Mupirocin-resistant MRSA transmission associated with community hospitals and nursing homes. J Hosp Infect 2010;75:141–2.

6. Mulvey MR, MacDougall L, Cholin B, et al, CA-MRSA Study Group. Community-associated methicillin-resistant *Staphylococcus aureus*, Canada. Emerg Infect Dis 2005;11:844–50.

7. Staidle JP, Benedetto AV, Benedetto PX, et al. Comparison of a novel antibiotic-free film-forming topical wound dressing versus triple antibiotic on Mohs surgical wounds 2018.

8. Sandhofer M, Schauer P. The safety, efficacy, and tolerability of a novel silicone gel dressing following dermatological surgery. Skinmed 2012;10(Suppl 1):S1–7.

9. Monk E, Benedetto E, Benedetto A. Successful treatment of nonhealing scalp wounds using a silicone gel. Dermatol Surg 2014;40:76–9.

10. Uva L, Aphale A, Kehdy J, et al. Erosive pustular dermatosis successfully treated with a novel silicone gel. Int J Dermatol 2016;55:89–91.

11. Marini L, Odendaal D, Smirnyi S. Importance of scar prevention and treatment: an approach from wound care principles. Dermatol Surg 2017;43:S85–90.

12. Non-Surgical Feminine Rejuvenation. The Aesthetic Guide. March/April 2017. Medical Insight. Available at: http://miinews.com/tag-archives/. Accessed April 1, 2018.

13. Nazarpour S, Simbar M, Tehrani FR. Factors affecting sexual function in menopause: a review article. Taiwan J Obstet Gynecol 2016;55:480–7.

14. Management of symptomatic vulvovaginal atrophy: 2013 position statement of the North American Menopause Society. Menopause 2013;20(9):888–902.

15. Lester J, Pahouja G, Andersen B, et al. Atrophic vaginitis in breast cancer survivors: a difficult survivorship issue. J Pers Med 2015;5(2):50–66. Available at: https://www.ncbi.nlm.nih.gov/pmc/articles/PMC4493485/.

16. Pauls R, Fellner AN, Davila GW. Vaginal laxity: a poorly understood quality of life problem; a survey of physician members of the International Urogynecological Association (IUGA). Int Urogynecol J 2012;23(10):1435–8.

17. Benedetto AV, editor. Botulinum toxins in clinical aesthetic practice, vol. 2, 3rd edition. Boca Raton (FL): CRC Press; 2018.

18. deAlmeida ART, Romiti A, Carruthers JDA. The facial platysma and its underappreciated role in lower face dynamics and contour. Dermatol Surg 2017;43(8):1042–9.

19. Botulinum Toxin Market Analysis By Type (Botulinum Toxin Type A, Botulinum Toxin Type B), By End Use (Therapeutic, Aesthetic), By Region (North America, Europe, Asia Pacific, Latin America, MEA), And Segment Forecasts, 2018–2025. GrandviewResearch.com. Available at: https://www.grandviewresearch.com/industry-analysis/botulinum-toxin-market. Accessed April 1, 2018.

20. Available at: https://www.aboutpharma.com/blog/2017/04/19/research-and-markets-global-botulinum-toxin-market-2013-2017-2025-major-players-are-allergan-ipsen-merz-medytox-us-worldmed-lanzhou-institute-of-biological-products-revance-therape/. Accessed April 1, 2018.

Moving?

Make sure your subscription moves with you!

To notify us of your new address, find your **Clinics Account Number** (located on your mailing label above your name), and contact customer service at:

Email: journalscustomerservice-usa@elsevier.com

800-654-2452 (subscribers in the U.S. & Canada)
314-447-8871 (subscribers outside of the U.S. & Canada)

Fax number: 314-447-8029

Elsevier Health Sciences Division
Subscription Customer Service
3251 Riverport Lane
Maryland Heights, MO 63043

*To ensure uninterrupted delivery of your subscription, please notify us at least 4 weeks in advance of move.

Printed and bound by CPI Group (UK) Ltd, Croydon, CR0 4YY

03/10/2024

01040298-0016